# Nature's Essential Oils

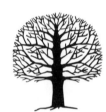

**THE COUNTRYMAN PRESS**
A division of W. W. Norton & Company
*Independent Publishers Since 1923*

# Nature's Essential Oils

**CHER KAUFMANN**

Aromatic
Alchemy
for Well-Being

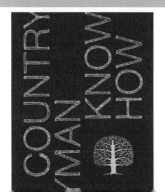

This volume is intended as a general information resource. It is not a substitute for medical advice. Essential oils can have or cause significant physical effects. If you have been diagnosed with, or suspect you may have, any medical or psychological condition, or if you are pregnant or considering pregnancy, consult your doctor or other professional healthcare provider before using essential oils. If you have questions about how to choose or use essential oils, consult an aromatherapist. Do not use essential oils to try to prevent illness, or in commercial settings. Be especially careful in using essential oils on or around babies, children, elderly people, and pets. Be sure to read the Author's Note for additional important safety guidelines.

References in this book to third-party organizations, tools, products and services are for general information purposes only. Neither the publisher nor the author can guarantee that any particular practice or resource will be useful or appropriate to the reader. Web addresses included in this book reflect links existing as of the date of first publication. The publisher is not responsible for the content of any website, blog or information page other than its own.

For information about permission to reproduce selections from this book,
write to Permissions, The Countryman Press 500 Fifth Avenue, New York, NY 10110

For information about special discounts for bulk purchases, please contact
W. W. Norton Special Sales at specialsales@wwnorton.com or 800-233-4830

Manufacturing by Versa Press
Series book design by Nick Caruso Design
Production manager: Devon Zahn

Library of Congress Cataloging-in-Publication Data

Names: Kaufmann, Cher, author.
Title: Nature's essential oils : aromatic alchemy for well-being / Cher Kaufmann.
Other titles: Aromatic alchemy for well-being
Description: New York, NY : The Countryman Press, A division of W.W. Norton & Company, [2018] |
    Series: Countryman know how | Includes bibliographical references and index.
Identifiers: LCCN 2018003692 | ISBN 9781581574593 (pbk. : alk. paper)
Subjects: LCSH: Essences and essential oils. | Essences and essential oils—Therapeutic use. | Odors—
    Psychological aspects. | Aromatherapy.
Classification: LCC QD416 .K2525 2018 | DDC 547/.71—dc23 LC record available at https://lccn.loc.gov/2018003692

The Countryman Press
www.countrymanpress.com

A division of W. W. Norton & Company, 500 Fifth Avenue, New York, NY 10110
www.wwnorton.com

978-1-58157-459-3 (pbk.)

10 9 8 7 6 5 4 3 2 1

## DEDICATION

To all those who are intrigued, who to want to know more, love to learn, and appreciate the profound magnitude of nature's cognizant power to sustain, teach, love, and know when to let go.

# AUTHOR'S NOTE

Making and using products with essential oils can bring you great peace, calm, and comfort. That's why I wrote this book. But essential oils are more than just relaxing scents. Essential oils have chemical properties that can affect you physically and emotionally. Even if you have the best of intentions, the use of essential oils can actually cause serious physical harm unless you know what you're doing, understand the risks, and follow the necessary safety rules. Also note that safety and usage recommendations are continually evolving.

The risks and rules are referenced throughout this book, not just in the sections that deal specifically with safety, but in the discussions of the chemistry of essential oils and the descriptions of the different kinds of individual oils. So, while it may be tempting to skip some parts and just get on to the recipes, PLEASE make sure you read and understand what the book says about:

- The importance of using pure essential oils
- How to identify pure essential oils
- The importance of always diluting essential oils in carrier oils
- How to use—and how not to use—essential oils
- When to use—and when not to use—essential oils
- When to give the body a rest from certain essential oils
- Potential allergic reactions to essential oils
- Phototoxic essential oils (which increase the risk of severe sunburn)
- The risks of using essential oils during pregnancy
- Using essential oils with children and babies
- Using essential oils with elderly people
- Using essential oils around pets
- Using minimum quantities (more does not equal better!)
- Proper dilution and dosages (see dilution and dosage charts)
- Maximum dilution for specific essential oils
- When not to use certain carrier oils
- Ensuring that store-bought ingredients are safe to use
- Sterilizing your essential oil containers
- Proper storage of your essential oil products
- The shelf life of different essential oil products

A few other key points that I want to address up front:

**DO NOT USE ESSENTIAL OILS IF . . . :** Even though many essential oils are safe for use by most people, to be on the safe side, I would recommend that essential oils not be used at all without a doctor's express permission for anyone who:

- Is pregnant
- Is nursing
- Is taking a prescription drug
- Is prone to seizures
- Has high blood pressure
- Is taking blood thinners
- Has a hormonal disorder
- Has estrogen-dependent cancer
- Has endometriosis
- Has any other diagnosed medical illness or condition

**DOCTORS vs. AROMATHERAPISTS:** It is crucial to understand when you need to consult a doctor and when you should consult an aromatherapist. If you think you may be physically or mentally ill, or if this book recommends using a particular essential oil to assist with a medical concern or condition, see your doctor or another professional healthcare provider for a medical diagnosis before using any essential oils. No aromatherapist can diagnose medical illness. But if you have questions about proper, safe use of essential oils, consult a qualified aromatherapist. Only qualified aromatherapists are trained in the chemistry and contraindications of essential oils and their appropriate, safe use. Many doctors have not been trained in aromatherapy, yet they add essential oils to their repertoire of remedies and make potentially unsafe recommendations—for example, telling patients to ingest essential oils or add undiluted drops to their bath water or skin. Make sure to ask questions and speak up if something doesn't make sense. Use an aromatherapist to learn how to use essential oils.

**WHO IS A BONA FIDE AROMATHERAPIST? :** A "qualified," "clinical," "trained," or "certified" aromatherapist is someone who has completed a formal clinical training program and has been certified by an association like the National Association for Holistic Aromatherapy (NAHA) and/or Alliance of International Aromatherapists (AIA). "Essential oil coaches," "wellness coaches," "wellness representatives," and sales representatives of multi-level marketing companies are NOT qualified aromatherapists.

**"PURE" OILS vs. IMITATION OILS:** Buyer beware! Less expensive essential oils from discount stores and online sellers may seem appealing, but they might be chemically adulterated and/or use falsified or old batch numbers to appear authentic. These oils, as well as synthetic oils and fragrance oils that are not pure essential oils, may contain no therapeutic value and may actually cause harm. Conversely, high

prices do not mean an oil is the "only" or "best" oil on the market. Many companies obtain oils from the same distilleries across the globe, thus no one company has the "only" source of oils. Research your sources, and ask an aromatherapist for a list of suggested essential oil retailers and educators. Find a few trusted sources rather than a single company. If you plan on making products using essential oils at home, only use authentic essential oils.

**ACTIVE vs. PREVENTATIVE:** Essential oils are not preventative. They are active substances. As soon as you apply an essential oil, whether you do it with a diffuser or in a cream or by any other delivery mechanism, that oil is acting on your body. Essential oils do not and cannot prevent illness or any particular condition any more than an antibiotic can prevent a virus. So, don't try to use them that way.

**DO NOT INGEST ANY ESSENTIAL OIL:** Do not ingest any essential oil or give any essential oil to someone else to ingest unless you have approval from your doctor and a clinical aromatherapist.

**NEVER USE OXIDIZED ESSENTIAL OILS:** Never use oxidized essential oils or essential oils that have exceeded their shelf life. They can irritate the skin.

**USING THE GLOSSARY AND INDEX:** Talking and teaching about essential oils involves a lot of technical terms. While I've tried to define each one the first time I use it, you can also find useful terms explained in the glossary. Don't assume you know what each of them means. Look it up in the index and then in the glossary.

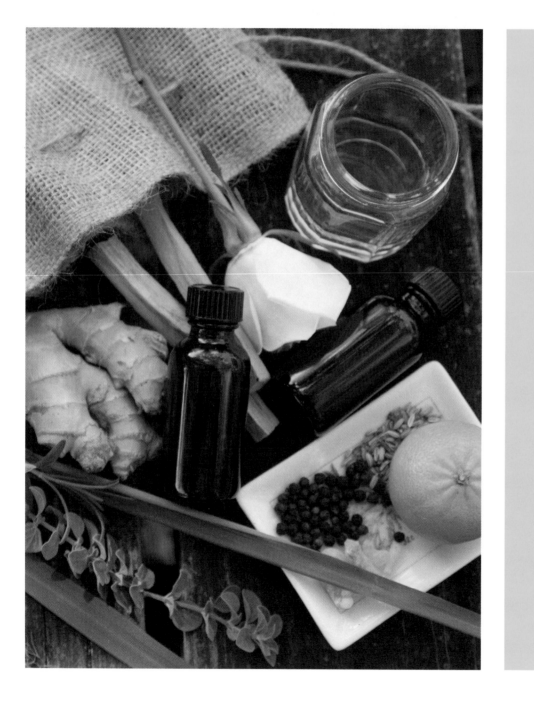

# CONTENTS

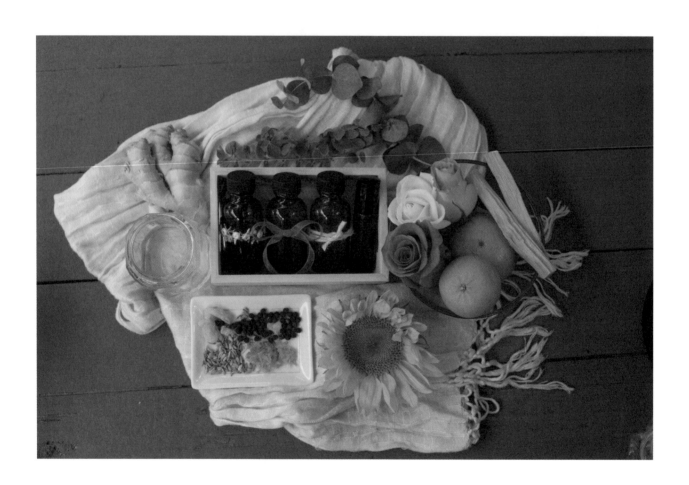

# Welcome

*Nature is ever at work building and pulling down, creating and destroying, keeping everything whirling and flowing, allowing no rest but in rhythmical motion, chasing everything in endless song out of one beautiful form into another.* —John Muir

Alchemy has always been a mysterious, magical, and mystical application of science mixed with experimentation and a lot of observation. Observation has been key to unlocking the connections between the thinking mind and the feeling heart. Noticing the change of seasons and nature's cyclical give-and-take has been the basis of entire cultures for thousands of years. Indian Ayurvedic, Traditional Chinese Medicine, and Arabic and Egyptian practices tap into alchemic powers.

For centuries, aromatic plants have been the source of many documented substances that promote beauty, health, and longevity. Essential oils, derived from these botanicals, are windows into those plants' energy, seductiveness, and survival, and connect us with an ancient consciousness that requires respect and observation to be fully understood. Still, knowledge of the alchemy of aromatherapy is in constant flux as more information is understood about the relationships between the natural world and humans. Truly dynamic topics are always expanding, and I hope that readers learn with anticipation of new discoveries and be mindful of the evolution of aromatic wonders. Welcome to the enchanting world of essential oils, the wisdom of nature, beyond the aroma.

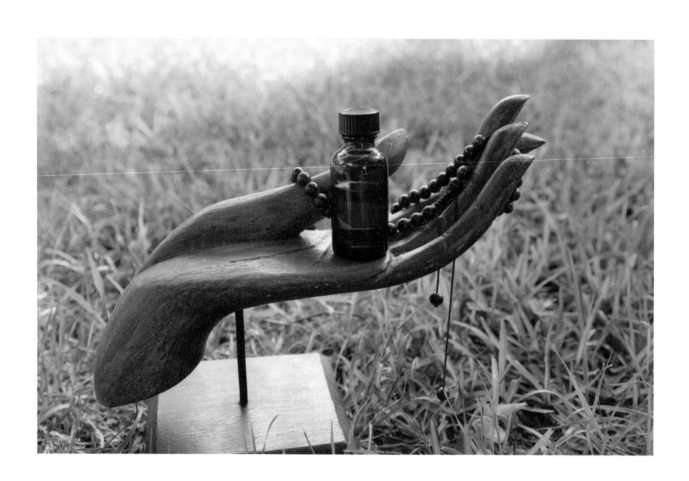

# Introduction

I used to skip the introductions of books. I figured I was going to learn the "real stuff" within the chapters. So, I can understand the appeal of jumping past the first steps. However, there is an important energetic sharing in an introduction.

Until recently, learning about essential oils usually involved searching in books, attending classes or workshops, or working one-on-one with someone knowledgeable in the subject. Now, with computers, the world is at our fingertips—yet that method of self-instruction does not always equate to safe, accurate information, nor the experiences gained in person or "real life." In this book, I make no assumptions that you already know about essential oils or use them. Essential oils are powerful and humble helpers to be used with honor and respect. The purpose of *Nature's Essential Oils* is to bring you closer to using these oils safely and with reverence.

This book is not designed to take you to an advanced level. If you are already familiar with essential oils, please use this as an opportunity to become better acquainted with them. Patience, eagerness, and a bit of curiosity are definitely first steps in learning something new. Consider this introduction a welcoming hand toward extending your knowledge.

In nature, certain plants produce essential oils to introduce themselves to the world, but it's not like a business meeting with a name tag that says, "Hi, my name is Plant." No, aromatic plants speak uniquely to the mind, body, and spirit of humans as well as to the other species on the planet. Those who jump past the basics, such as where particular plants grow, or even what part of a plant is used to obtain an oil, are missing out on important knowledge.

Our world is very sensory; our body, also. Every bit of sensory information provides us with visual, emotional, mental, and spiritual intelligence. Just as the passing breeze tugging at your clothes or whishing through your hair as you stand on your porch comes from the same air system ultimately responsible for waves on a beach, our world is intimately connected: it overlaps, intertwines, and exchanges with a constant giving and receiving of atoms. This happens each time you apply aromatherapy to your life. Knowing more about the plant-derived material that you are putting on your skin or breathing into your lungs, which ultimately enters your body and your brain, can be helpful in understanding its effects.

Essential oils have quite a history, but not as long as the use of aromatic plants in general. Learning more about these botanicals enriches your knowledge and honors an ecological system of natural resources, some of which are in danger of being overharvested. When introduced with care, essential oils are wonderful tools that anyone can use responsibly and share with others safely. When some steps are skipped, or essential oils are used incorrectly, the results can be disappointing, expensive, and possibly damaging.

In the beginning, take the time to get to know a few essential oils really well and they will serve you in many ways. You will have a better handle on what to use in a time of crisis, rather than trying to look up something from a list of 300-plus possibilities. Think of it as having several good friends you know you can count on when you need them most. In this book, I will suggest some great beginner oils, but you will discover your own "top 10" list as you become more familiar with oils and your family's needs.

Take the time to read and reread at your own pace. Think of this journey as your introduction to a much bigger picture without your having to know all of it at one time. The more you see the different facets of essential oils, like a prism of light, the more confidently and safely you can express the rainbow of possibilities in your choices. Be open to learning new things and they will teach you about yourself and the world around you in wonderful ways.

## My Introduction to Essential Oils

I long have been curious about subjects that have not always fallen into mainstream knowledge, such as theology, quantum physics, Ayurveda, and Traditional Chinese Medicine. I am inquisitive, yes, but really I am intrigued. I genuinely want to know more about my fellow humans and the world around me.

My first introduction to essential oils was in my late teens and early twenties in the late 1980s and early '90s, when I became curious about the interesting things sold in small health food stores. But the oils and I only made eye contact back then; I never really got to know them by name. After college, I spent the next 20 years in alternative health care, studying everything from Reiki, massage therapy, and Chinese face reading to energetic healing modalities and patterns in people, before becoming an author and inspirational art instructor, teaching about the fantastical world of patterns.

While I was in massage school in the mid- to late 1990s, we were encouraged to experiment in classes and internships with different lotions and creams. This was my second introduction to essential oils. Many students combined the oils whose scent they liked. I remember one classmate who always mixed rosemary and lavender together based solely on smell, not because of their properties. And, of course, there was always someone who opted for a heady, sweet, artificial vanilla scent (whew! I remember it well!). I don't recall anyone counting how many drops we added to our lotions; then, we used a plastic bottle's pump mechanism to mix the oils the best we could or shook the lotion until we thought it was mixed. Or until it "smelled" mixed. No exact science involved. There was no formal instruction—for us, scented oils were just options to "enhance" a massage.

When I reflect back, I am embarrassed at how nonchalantly I had treated the oils, because I consider myself to be pretty aware of the overall connection between things. But at that time, I was more focused on the actual massage and energetic exchange between the client and myself. Essential oils, to my inexperienced mind, were simply a nice thing to add. They smelled good. They did stuff. At least, that was what we were told. Using them made us feel professional. Making things smell good has been in practice for thousands of years, right? Wasn't that what the oils were for? It was all so vague. And superficial. One thing I remember from those days

and many years afterward was I was not a fan of lavender or rose. I wonder now whether somehow I knew what I was smelling then was not the real deal. Artificially scented rose and lavender lotions had been on the market for a long time, because genuine oils can be expensive. But once you smell the real thing—it's worth every cent.

I gained employment at a massage therapy supply store while going to massage school and remained there for a time after I acquired my licensed massage therapist credentials. The store carried essential oils, and with some authority I would sell them easily because I repeated what was told to me by my employers. Plus, I would read the information on the bottles, memorizing which oil matched the description of what the person was looking for: "Lavender: calming, relaxing" or "Lemon: uplifting, stimulating." While my basic information was correct, and technically I was steering everyone in the right direction, an indispensable piece was missing.

I was curious enough to acquire a small library of essential oil books over the years and attended classes taught by various aromatherapy teachers, herbalists, and alternative health educators. I used my knowledge to suggest essential oils for family members, friends, and clients, and applied the oils in my massage therapy practice. Yet book knowledge and taking classes does not equal wisdom. Over time, I certainly understood much more about essential oils than did the average consumer, but I still did

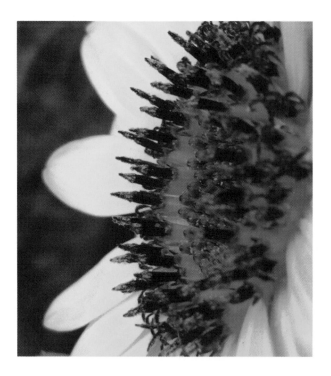

not feel I really knew the oils. Something was still missing.

My third introduction to essential oils occurred several years prior to my aromatherapy certification. I've always loved studying patterns. I notice things, things people overlook or choose not to see. I feel shifts in energy patterns when someone's emotions change inside. I can feel physical heat or tingling patterns off a body when something is going on within it. I observe natural phenomena, such as the way sunflowers, when viewed from the side, appear to have eyelashes thick with mascara before the inner seed center develops. People, places, sounds, and objects have a certain color or "feel" to me that is sometimes hard to explain with words. Even numbers show up for me in particular patterns (every single time). My observation of how resistant certain plants are to being uprooted and how others give up their space in the dirt so easily, tells me a lot about their relative steadfastness. It is really the same as observing people when they shyly move out of the way for others or "dig in their heels" and refuse to budge.

These are not "way out" sensations reserved for the strange and unusual or psychic. They are actually what other creatures and plants experience—an awareness of the environment and subtle changes that happen within our surroundings. Animals can sense earthquakes before they happen; insects detect changes in light, temperature, and odor to find the best source of food. Plants can anticipate grazing animals' habits and release chemicals that change their flavor, making them less palatable, ensuring at least some of the plants survive and thrive. We are all part of nature and have natural abilities to connect to the world. Many, though, are either told not to listen to the communication of their body, much less that of other species, or perhaps just not encouraged to listen. I often wonder whether synchronicity is simply good listening—not just through the ears, but with the entire body, mind, and spirit.

My later introduction to essential oils was unlike

my previous casual experiences. I think the right teacher appears when the student is ready. This time, I was ready to pay attention to the oils as they connect to nature, not just as liquid in a bottle. This time, I met them with an open heart, respecting and honoring the power of the plants, the soil, the sun and moon. It was what gardeners feel when they really get to know a plant, or how an animal lover intuitively connects with a fluffy pet, knowing so much with just an ear flicker. More to the point, I had not known what I was missing until I took the time to really become acquainted. This time, the oils introduced themselves, sharing information I had overlooked for years. This time, I listened.

When I heard it, the rise and fall of each oil's song was a breath from the universe of botanical wonders, a giving and receiving from the essential oil, the plant, and the earth to me. Essential oils speak through the aromatic molecules in hints and whispers of flowers through the heavy scent of fallen rain and the soft warmth of rooted seclusion. Once the art of aromatherapy had finally been exposed to me, much like a strong beam of light shining through a cluster of clouds, I not only knew facts about plants, I could *feel* them.

Since then, I have deepened my experiences by distilling wild harvested trees and plants in the southwest summer Arizonan desert, listening to each tree as I touched its branches, able to sense that some trees were stronger than others, their fragrance and essential oils reflecting this energy.

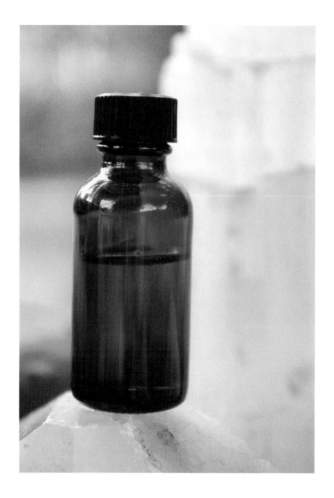

Instead of sitting in classrooms, I have traveled around the country, visiting botanical and organic gardens, interviewing aromatherapists and master herbalists, and chatting with master gardeners.

At home, I have added herbs, spices, and flowering plants back into my neglected garden space.

Nature's cycle of growing, adapting, releasing, and dying reflects so much of our human nature. Nature is powerful. It is also very subtle. Do not be too surprised if your interest in the natural world begins to take on a new meaning once you develop your knowledge of essential oils.

## Stress Relief Smells Good

Essential oils are much more than a matched ailment and solution in a chart for headaches or ant bites, albeit some charts can be valuable while one is learning. The essences of plants, flowers, trees, resins, and more are living energies that we respond to biologically, emotionally, mentally, and spiritually. Although independent essential oil scientist Dr. Robert Pappas would argue that anything that goes through the temperatures of a distillation process is technically no longer alive, something biocompatible and active is still very much present in essential oils.

Our body and mind relate viscerally to the stimulation of our senses. The smell of pine or fir stimulates a deeper breath and images of a forest. In the invisible world of essential oils, healing responses occur where biological harmony is created. Truth is, smelling things you like will reduce stress! Even just deep breaths reduce stress.

In England, one of the tenets of education for aromatherapy has always been from a place of

Using essential oils is not the same thing as diagnosing people's medical conditions. No one except a licensed medical doctor can diagnose. However, you can learn to be observant to the needs of the body, mind, emotions, and spirit, which varies according to the individual. Pay attention to how you or your family reacts to the stress-reducing support of particular essential oils. For example, frustrations and anger do well with calming oils, such as lavender or citruses; whereas if you need a clear head to study or work on a project, try upbeat aromas, such as rosemary, plus creative support, such as palo santo.

stress relief. This is immeasurably different than diagnostic treatment, which only happens in clinical settings. An aromatherapist's goal is to create health and harmony with gentleness, avoiding any possible harmful action. The retailers who have been bitten by the commercial product bug sometimes forget that many factors go into using essential oils.

Understanding sustainability (these oils are, after all, from living aspects of the planet), which often translates to less is more, plus respecting their power and safe usage, are key to a sound experience as you begin exploring the world of essential oils. With the increase in information accessibility comes the importance to discern between sharing information and *advising* or *diagnosing*. That is, holding or attending a home party based around essential oils does not make you an aromatherapist, just as being a regular customer at a restaurant does not make you a chef. Diagnosis is not within the scope of any home user. Stress relief, however, is! Be sure to read Part 2 on safety as it is very important on your aromatic journey.

So, make a cup of tea, find a relaxing place, take a deep breath, and begin reading. Nature welcomes you to participate in this discussion with nature's ancient alchemy.

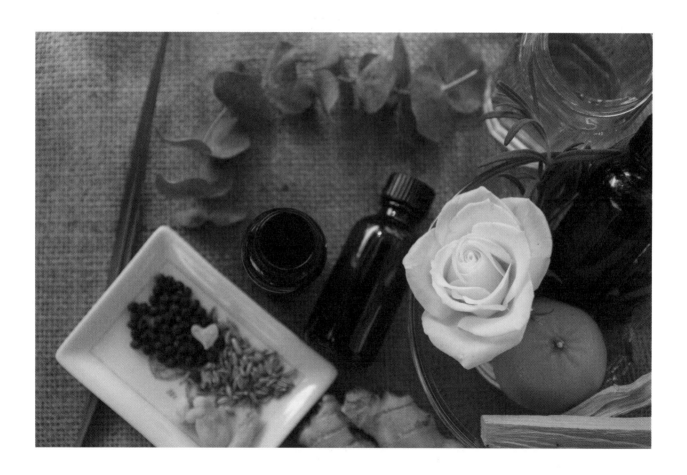

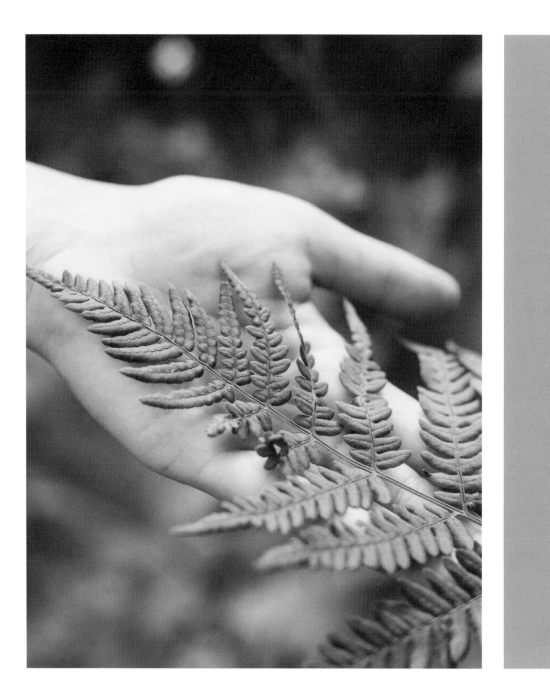

# Nature

1

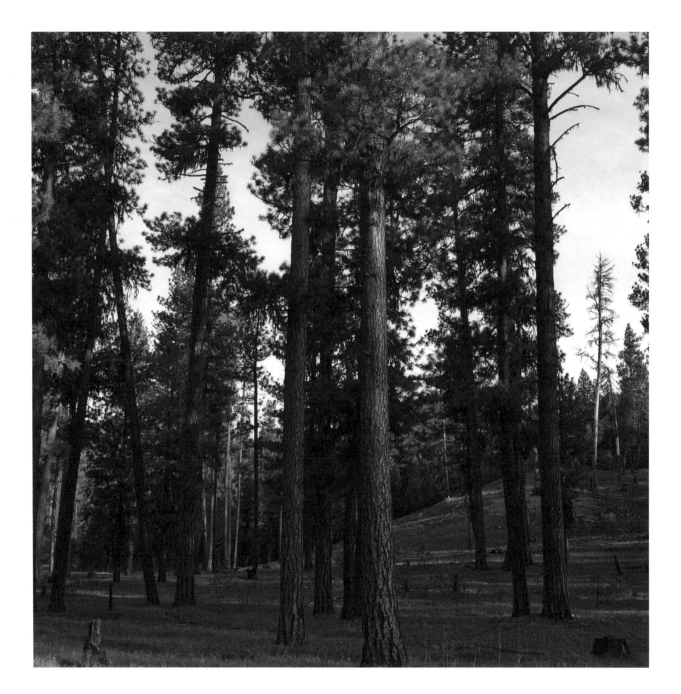

# The Natural World

*I care to live only to entice people to look at Nature's loveliness.* —John Muir

The scenery had changed dramatically from the dry desert mountains and mostly brown landscape of southern Nevada as my family and I headed back to Texas from a long road trip. Now, while we drove in late afternoon through the lush, green ponderosa pines in the Coconino National Forest in northern Arizona, the scent of pine poured in through our open windows, a gentle wave of aroma flooding the car, permeating our hair and our clothes. The deep breaths we all took were intentional, as we tried to gather in as much as we could of this seemingly otherworldly divine forest presence.

When you inhale the scent of a forest, you are taking in its phytoncides present in the air—the volatile vapors released from the trees, whose purpose appears to be to activate immunity for the whole forest community by triggering purification of the air and providing air ionization. The clean, clear air refreshes and boosts the brain and body function of forest creatures (or visiting humans), who in return breathe out carbon dioxide, necessary for plant survival. Phytoncides are, in essence, "the influence of higher plants on microorganisms" and their activity "is conditioned by the species of the plant, its age, growth stage and intensity of photosynthesis and also depends on climatic and soil environmental conditions" (Waksmundzka-Hajnos and Sherma 2010). That is to say, they are antimicrobial: they kill microbes naturally. These compounds have been studied in natural forest settings and by diffusing essential oils of pine and cypress, to measure their influence on the human body. In each case, human natural killer (NK) cells increased and stress hormone levels decreased (Li, et al. 2009). That is, the health of the tree benefits the health of the forest; the health of the forest, in turn, supports the health of humans.

Forest bathing, known as *shinrin-yoku* ("taking

in the forest atmosphere") in Japan, has been shown to boost the immune system by increasing the count of natural killer (NK) cells, reducing blood pressure and stress, improving mood and focus, and increasing energy level and improving sleep (Park, et al. 2010). The practice of spending time in natural settings for health benefits is becoming better known as urban living decreases activity in and the availability of such settings. With the deep breath of forest air, especially a forest of pines, there are striking results, some lasting for up to a month after a weekend of exposure to the trees (Li, et al. 2009). But not all plants release natural vapors into the air to support the community of an entire ecosystem. That is what makes aromatic plants amazing, and aromatic trees so important.

Only a small percentage of plants on the planet can change the air quality, fragrance, and health of the world through scent. I can't help but wonder whether the delicate balance of having just the right amount of organisms functioning in this way ensures that all other creatures are not bombarded with an overload of odors. This scarcity allows all species to distinguish and take notice when aromatic changes are present in the environment. Historically, such plants developed scent even before they did color. There is evidence that they know what they are doing when the scent is released. Their reactions to environmental changes in the air or to attacks by insects or herbivores, or their invitation for pollinators to come a little closer, are all intentional chemical changes for the survival and

*Phyto*, meaning "plant" or "relating to plants," derives from the Greek *phuton* ("plant") and *phuein* ("come into being"); *-cide* means "kill."

enticement of the plant. Their essential oils are valuable to our sense of smell and physical, mental, emotional, and spiritual connections to plants in general.

## A (Short) History of Aromatic Plants

In brief, essential oils are volatile substances produced through a series of chemical processes, beginning with the energy from the sun, which assist the protection and reproduction of a plant. They are not necessary for plants to survive, otherwise all plants would have essential oils. Normal growth and development is not affected by the production or presence of essential oils. They are, in fact, secondary metabolites, whereas primary metabolites are components necessary to plant growth and development, such as amino acids and carbohydrates. Only 10% of the entire plant kingdom produce these volatiles. Those that do are often called aromatic plants. They contain specific components with particular purposes. Lavender and rose are obviously aromatic plants, but sometimes hidden parts of plants, such as the roots of vetiver grass or ginger rhizomes, also contain an essential oil.

People are usually introduced to essential oils in a way that captivates their sense of smell. They relax if the aroma is pleasant and perk up if the scent is crisp. Perhaps this is what first drew humans to investigate certain plants for eating, healing, or burning—say, the scent of certain woods in a fire or a sweet fragrance of ripe fruit. Whatever the enticement was in the very beginning, it worked. Plants found a way to communicate their many potential purposes, including sustaining their own longevity and health, from which humans have benefited, in the form of plant-derived food, drink, shelter, tools, and more. Aromatic plants, however, have extra powers, such as healing wounds (lavender), purifying the air (pine), flavoring food (lemon), or assisting with meditation (frankincense) or embalming (cedarwood).

The uses of aromatic plants have largely predated their documentation in recorded history, although there are mentions in ancient texts. Egyptians in 3500 BC, Greeks in 1100–140 BC, and Romans from the tenth century to around AD 1453 all used aromatic plants and their extractions. Cleopatra lured Mark Antony and Julius Caesar into her affections with what is thought to have been her heavy use of scented cones of wax that would melt, anointing her with perfume. Egyptians quite possibly had the most complex early understanding of aromatics from their use with mummification, perfumed adornments, and vessels containing remnants in tombs of pharaohs, but they certainly were not the first.

Volatile organic compounds change from a liquid to a vapor easily and have a molecular carbon base. Carbon molecules are found in all living organisms, making them biochemically recognizable by other living beings. The volatile liquid-to-vapor organic compounds of plant substances used in aromatherapy are essential oils.

The Rigveda, an Indian text from 5000 BC predating documents of the Egyptians, records 67 medicinal plants. Ayurveda, an Indian philosophy and lifestyle that predates Christianity, and which is based on seasonal rotation of nature for food and well-being, made heavy use of aromatic plants, herbs, and medicated oils. Medicated oils are specific concoctions created by cooking herbs and aromatic plants in oils for the purpose of massaging the body, certainly a precursor to the anointment with oils used in many religions.

Aromatic plants have been used for scent and the easing of ailments for thousands of years. The choice of the aromas and properties of the plants chosen for such mixtures changed over time. These mixtures were crude perfumes, but certainly people understood that certain combinations worked better than others.

The Bible mentions fragrant resins of frankincense and myrrh, and it is speculated that turmeric was the "gold" brought by the Wise Men to the baby Jesus. Traditional Chinese Medicine, thought to

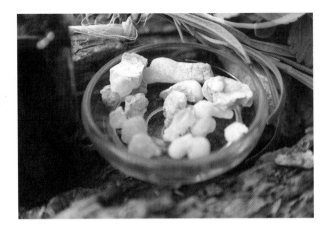

have developed shortly after Ayurveda, employed certain spices, aromatic herbs, and other plants as a means to unstick and harmonize qi, the vital force in the body. Spices from aromatic plants, used in trade and as currency, show just how incredibly valuable these treasures of nature have been in the journey of human exploration of the planet. The Silk Road was an active trade route between China and the Mediterranean for not only silk but spices, herbs, and aromatics from the second century BC to the end of the fourteenth century.

Scent is but one of many attributes of essential oils. Historically, aromatic plants themselves have been made into tinctures, used as flavorings for food and drink, placed in fire pits or slow-burning embers for purifying, and smoked. Utilizing aromatic plants and resins during religious ceremonies has served not only to produce a calming connection to the meditative states of ritual, but also as a practical means of combatting pathogens in the air. According to herbalist, acupuncturist, and aromatherapist David Crow, burning aromatic plants during ceremonies helped keep the smell of body odor down, purified the air when a population congregated in close quarters, and kept a calm, centered mind of those gathered. Plus, an association between the scent and the purpose of the ritual became imprinted in the psyche of all who attended.

It has been widely accepted that during the Middle Ages, in the times of the plague, the use of aromatic plants was key to maintaining the health of many people. Doctors would place a combination of herbs and aromatic plants in a long, beaklike air filter that they would wear over their face and head, to protect themselves. The famous stories of four thieves who would loot homes of the sick and gravesites of the deceased, yet somehow staving off disease, goes back to a mixtures of herbs and vinegar they used on their body and clothes. French doctor and aromatherapist Jean Valnet (1920–1995) turned up a few recipes of these infamous mixtures in the archives of the Parliament of Toulouse. The recipes have some differences, but the consistent appearance of certain aromatic herbs and spices, such as rosemary, sage, and cloves, does lean toward what science now knows about their antibacterial and antiseptic properties. Even Hippocrates, a Greek physician who used aromatic plants for medicinal purposes, was a big fan of daily aromatic baths and scented massages. There really is no place in history where aromatics were not used in some way.

Historically, the crude distillation of aromatic

plants in rudimentary stills can be traced as far back as 3000 BC. Ancient cultures in Egypt, India, and China had detailed knowledge of how to create perfumes and oils from plants, along with using them for medicines and herbal remedies. Wines and alcohol are documented as having been used in libation ceremonies across continents for thousands of years. Aromatic waters, known as flower waters or hydrolats, were long used for cooking, toilet waters, perfumes, and baths. In fact, these distilled waters have a longer recorded history than do essential oils as we know them. Herbal infusions from the plants were made using thick oils, honey, or fats, yes, but essential oils as a stand-alone distilled substance did not exist until very recently.

This is not because essential oils were not used (they are, after all, part of an aromatic plant and would naturally be present in any use of such plants), but because distillation for the sole purpose of extracting an essential oil was not taking place. It took an Arabic child prodigy, Avicenna (ca. 980–1037), to fine-tune the distillation process, improving the cooling system with the invention of a refrigeration coil, which allowed temperatures to separate the water from the essential oils. Avicenna distilled the first essential oil: rose. This small shift changed the path of future essential oils to be possible and purposefully crafted.

However, centuries passed until pure essential oils were what distillers were looking for—what they wanted was distilled flower waters. Certainly, mentions of essential oil use were documented by

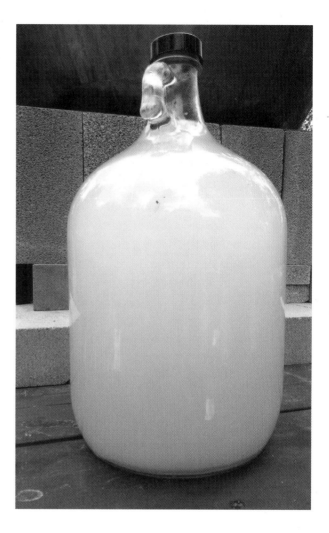

Nicholas Culpeper, the famous herbalist, botanist, and physician, in the 1600s. Uses are also listed in pharmaceutical dispensary references in the late 1800s and early 1900s. When French perfumer and scientist René-Maurice Gattefossé documented

scientific research on the subject in the early 1900s, interest began in the beneficial health effects of specific essential oils, beyond perfumery. He was the first to figure out how to remove some of the harsher chemical constituents and to make lavender usable for scent soaps.

Intentional distillation for essential oils, as we refer to them now in modern aromatherapy, is often credited to the twentieth century, when they were used for medicinal purposes and sold by traditional pharmacies in Europe to practitioners for therapeutic purposes only, unavailable to the general public.

## The Modern World

*Aromatherapie* was originally coined in 1937 by Gattefossé, who began to teach distillation, study, and document essential oils as relating to therapeutic uses. This changed the way essential oils were looked at—as distinct from perfumery alone. He obtained some of his information from villagers who shared with him utilization of plants in specific ways for healing wounds. The most infamous legend about Gattefossé was a lab explosion, which he described in his 1937 book *Aromatherapie* as follows:

> The external application of small quantities of essences rapidly stops the spread of gangrenous sores. In my personal experience, after a laboratory explosion covered me with burning substances which I extinguished by rolling on a grassy lawn, both my hands were covered with a rapidly developing gas gangrene. Just one rinse with lavender essence stopped "the gasification of the tissue." This treatment was followed by profuse sweating, and healing began the next day (July 1910). (Tisserand blogpost 2011)

Robert Tisserand explains that this incident was not what sparked (literally) Gattefossé's study of essential oils, since this application of lavender was clearly intentional, based in knowledge Gattefossé had picked up from his perfumery and botany studies abroad. However, it did serve as one of the many stepping-stones in his journey toward documenting and collaborating with others on the study of essential oils, especially their antibacterial and anti-inflammatory benefits. This important moment in history begins to pave the way to the essential oil understanding as we know it today (Tisserand 2011).

Jean Valnet published *The Practice of Aromatherapy* in 1964, in France. Much of his work consisted in documenting and teaching essential oils usage safely—with the *maximum benefit* and *minimum risk of harm*. Dr. Valnet created several essential oil–based antiseptic remedies during World War II. His contribution to making essential oils viable options in medical settings and for wound care expanded the study to what is now French aromatherapy. Another contributor to the advance of the therapeutic uses of essential oils was Marguerite Maury, born in Austria in 1895, who worked in Vienna and France as a nurse and emphasized a holistic approach, always considering the *well-being of the whole, rather than the parts of a person*. Maury used touch, such as aromatherapy massage, to administer the gentle and powerful effects of essential oils through the skin, using diluted lotions and oils.

Since the turn of the twentieth century, France has been a vital part of the modern connection to plant-based products, including herbal oils and teas developed for beauty and health, and has long been considered the lavender capital of the world. France's growing conditions, soil, and altitude are particularly supportive to a sublime crop of lavender. However, due to climate change in the early twenty-first century, which is causing warmer temperatures at higher altitudes and pests, such as cicadas, growers of the famous lavender of Provence have had to reevaluate the growing area. Moving to higher altitudes closer to the mountains, to capture the ancient balance of weather and survival, has been the solution to accommodate for human city growth and development. It is also thought that the heat produced from the larger cities may be having an effect of the pristine temperatures perfect for the French lavender. Hence, Bulgaria has become a primary lavender supplier in a time of France's crop issues.

Some aromatherapists still active in the holistic aromatherapy industry have been part of the community since the 1970s and '80s. Back then, information (on any subject, skill, or art form) had

Marguerite Maury's contributions to aromatherapy were very holistic:

- Using massage with essential oils to increase the absorption, relaxing effects, and overall beneficial results, instead of using massage alone. This became known as integrative massage with essential oils, or aromatherapy massage.
- Looking beyond a physical ailment to include emotional concerns and mental stresses—in other words, at the whole person—is just as important when considering the right blend for an individual. Nutrition, hydrotherapy, exercise, and other therapies should also be considered for a complete balanced approach—not just essential oils alone. This became a very important part of the holistic approach used today.
- One size does not fit all. Individual considerations of all the parts that make each person unique are emphasized in the holistic approach. One essential oil may not be the best approach for someone's neighbor, same as an exercise routine or nutrient requirements.
- Every oil is multifaceted. Observation of the psychological and physical benefits of an essential oil are equally valued. The mental and emotional benefits can have a direct result on the physical. As a matter of fact, when stress is high, the sensation of pain tends to increase. Use the appropriate relaxation properties of each oil to assist in well-being.

to be purposely sought after. The age of technology was not digital and serious students and inquisitive persons would gather personal experiences by being introduced to the specific field of study. Ideas were shared in person or by way of carefully organized pamphlets, workbooks, and published books. Classes were experiential: students touched, smelled, connected with the essential oils and the plants from which they came, and learned from hands-on guidance in the fields and gardens of growers. In the case of essential oils, a small group (by today's standards) of curious minds shared enough information that soon a group of educators blossomed in the United States by the 1990s to share information from Europe and other countries.

After a while, all the educators had mostly been introduced to one another and a soft lull gently blanketed the industry. The work continued quietly. Everyone had shared with others as much as possible whatever information was available, ranging from folklore to anecdotal evidence to scientific or medical fact. It was not until the 1980s, but even more so into the 1990s, that the retail market for essential oils really took off, especially when educated professional aromatherapists and the general public in the United States alike had access to these oils. Even so, in the 1970s, '80s, and '90s, only those who were previously familiar with the oils or who frequented health food stores or maintained holistic health practices kept essential oils alive in the retail market. Aromatherapists emerged, oftentimes with herbalism or another form of alternative health

## MYTH: ESSENTIAL OILS CAN HELP WITH EVERYTHING (A.K.A. "THERE'S AN OIL FOR THAT.").

Essential oils are very powerful, yet can be equally subtle, gentle, and comforting. Sometimes oils are not the best match for what is going on. Instead, the best way to relieve whatever stress is presenting itself might be by drinking tea, turning on a fan and clearing the air, taking a nap, or trying another form of holistic health care, such as massage therapy, acupuncture, or chiropractic. Or it might be getting lab work from your medical practitioner. Nutrition and exercise might need some attention and essential oils might be additional helpers for support. Essential oils are helpful, but they are only one of *many* amazing options in creating a supportive health network for your well-being. Choose wisely and appropriately what works best for individual situations. There is always more than one way, but rarely only one way.

care as an overlap in their repertoire, such as massage therapy or acupuncture. It was a community of understanding nature and holistic health care. The mind-set came from a place of deep insights, accumulating nuggets of wisdom, and establishing a trove of intuitive and empirical knowledge a little at a time.

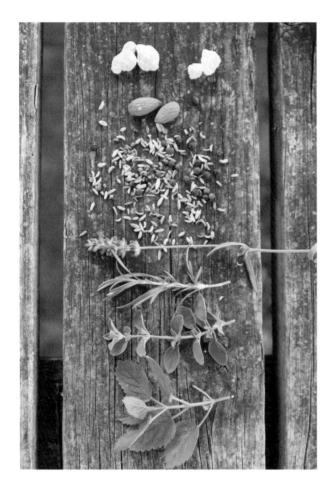

well-being with a holistic approach. Retail companies discovered many ways to market essential oils. Although making the oils available to nonprofessional home users was not new, a critical piece was now missing, compared with the educational process of previous years: instead, science and technology suddenly jumped ahead of users' slow-paced, gentle, experiential introduction to essential oils, to a fast-tracked end product. This created a boom in interest in essential oils as a merchandise unit, but not necessarily in the art of aromatherapy as a trained practice. While pioneers of the industry, like Kurt Schnaubelt, Jane Buckle, and Jeanne Rose, were sharing information with professionals in the field, newcomers often overlooked these experts as resources.

This led to the development of an important part of essential oil education: consumer protection. Robert Tisserand and Rodney Young published the second edition of *Essential Oil Safety*, and scientists, such as Dr. Robert Pappas and others, began testing oils for adulterations as a call to educate aromatherapists and essential oil enthusiasts on the power, interactions, precautions, and values of individual oils. Clinical aromatherapy with intensive chemistry instruction deepened the curriculum through the work of instructors such as Mark Webb and Dr. Timothy Miller. Madeleine Kerkhof-Knapp Hayes taught palliative care using supercritical extracted oils ($CO_2$s), as well steam-extracted essential oils in Europe and America, further broadening the scope of mindful and careful applications. Their

Then, 25 to 30 years into the mainstream essential oil industry, a shift occurred that changed education and usage: technology. A new wave of commerce boomed quickly. Clever footholds in creating multilevel marketing to reach more people became a much different approach, one much more businesslike, than the original intent to create

work produced waves in the aromatherapy world of which was the "right" way to proceed with education and the industry as a whole.

With the advent of the Internet, aromatherapy became mainstream and popular, but with a downside: without herbal, holistic, or even basic aromatherapy training, improper and hazardous use and advice of essential oils was spreading rapidly. Children, adults, and pets began experiencing adverse reactions to the haphazard use of these oils. In response, educators created online education, in-person classes, and books, providing more options to gain training than had been the case for many years. This was to meet the demands of a technology-savvy audience that was often gathering erroneous, sometimes even dangerous, advice with little regard to proper safety and precautions. But good has come of this: the creation for more mindful approaches in education, accountability as to who is teaching what, and increased understanding of which oils are suitable for aromatherapy versus to create pleasant scents. Increased testing, labeling, and clarifications of plant properties have moved to the forefront in education as well as in product development.

Essential oils are at the exact moment in history when people just like you are seeking natural health, well-being, and home solutions for family and loved ones. Serious students of aromatherapy are now reexamining what they thought they knew, or at the very least, cross-referencing their sources. Curious minds that are not serious students of the subject,

*Adulteration* is when an essential oil has been altered with filler oils or chemical compositions to mimic a smell, but it does not have the phytochemistry of the original plant, making it void of therapeutic value. Robert Pappas is an independent chemist who specializes in testing for pure essential oils and the telltale chemical markers that show whether an oil has been changed intentionally. Dr. Pappas uses equipment in his lab to prove authenticity as well as to uncover false claims made by certain companies selling to the public, a process called GC/MS testing (see page 62).

who are getting their botanical information easily and superficially, often using social media as a main source of information, may be having some unfortunate experiences. Sometimes it takes being introduced to the subject from several sources, as well as searching for credible authorities, to gain a more harmonized approach.

## Nature Speaks through Essential Oils

Returning to the road trip among the Coconino National Forest, with its soft allure of ponderosa pines, there was a desire to pull over to one of the picnic areas. We all got out and looked up at the towering trees, somehow feeling and sensing the unseen yet palpable blanket of soothing calm in the area. Everything felt connected here—the undergrowth, the birds, and the trees. David George Haskell, author of *The Songs of Trees*, reminds us that we are not separate from nature—as if nature itself was some outside mysterious force, and we, an illusionary philosophically detached "other"—rather, "our bodies and minds, our 'Science and Art' are as natural and wild as they ever were."

Nature's perseverance is a constant rise and fall: its breath, its flow of fluids, its sharing with multiple species in exchanges encountered in passing, even its permanence, as with the soil. According to scientists at Umeå University, Sweden is home to the longest-living organism, a Norway spruce called Old Tjikko, which has been cloning itself for more than nine millennia. "Spruce trees can multiply with the root penetrating branches to produce the exact copies of themselves, so while the individual trunk is younger, the organism has been cloning itself for at least 9,550 years" (Goldbaum 2016). The essential oil of the black spruce, a different species but same genus, lessens adrenal fatigue. Not always recognized as a medical condition, adrenal fatigue is when a person has been using his or her inner resources (mental, emotional, or physical), not resting nor rejuvenating appropriately, depleting the natural cortisol levels produced by the adrenal glands to cope with stress. To assist the body by another species that

seems to know a thing or two about long-term pacing and survival is a bridge of natural biochemistry. A sharing of natural wisdom.

## Homeopathic Essences vs. Essential Oils

Homeopathy works on the idea of "like cures like," looking for mirroring indicators to reflect back to the body that it is out of harmony in a particular way. Similarly, flower essences, originally developed by Edward Bach, an English homeopath, use the subtle energetics of flowers to assist the mental and emotional properties of the human experience. Whereas homeopathy and flower essences use no external sensory input, other than taking the remedies, essential oils use multiple senses to engage a variety of organs to stimulate the homeostasis every human body strives for each day. Some of the same plants are used in both practices; for example, hypericum (known as St. John's wort in the herbal world), a homeopathic essence, is also used in aromatherapy as an herbal infused oil. Just as nature uses multiple avenues to give you clean water, great air, nourishing foods, and medicines, essential oils are one of many natural, beautiful avenues provided in cooperation between the plants and humans.

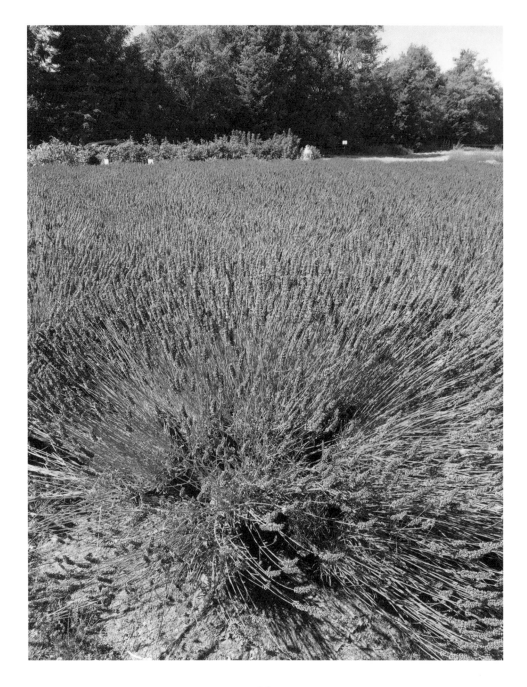

# CHAPTER 2

# What's in the Bottle?

*When we tug at a single thing in nature, we find it attached to the rest of the world.* —John Muir

Hold it up to the light and the liquid inside an amber or cobalt blue bottle pretty much looks like any other. But this magic elixir is the end product of a series of events. Surprisingly many people, including those already familiar with essential oils, do not know how an oil is produced, nor from which plants they come. Equally stunning is how few are aware that the sun and the moon, where a plant is grown, and when it was harvested all affect the potency of an essential oil. This is what one of my mentors, herbalist/aromatherapist David Crow, meant when he asked, "What's in the bottle?" Those simply using essential oils from a bottle, with no thought to where they come from, are woefully disconnected from the magic of nature's gifts.

As humans, complex and intricate, our six senses are integral in communication to our inner being (organs, hormones, emotions, and physical functions) and outer being (environment). The obvious five senses of sight, sound, taste, touch, and smell are what we rely on to provide information from the world around us. The sixth sense is an often underused sense of intuition, or that gut feeling, as it were. It is an important sense to mention, because even though science is unable to measure it in the same fashion as the other senses, if you ask any scientists who are really good at their job, they will tell you somewhere along the way they've conducted experiments or achieved results based on a hunch, or a feeling, or a sense of unseen direction. Even other species on the planet exhibit a "knowing" to unseen changes in environment.

## Plant Smarts

To understand essential oils, it is helpful, and in some ways necessary, to understand plants. Those

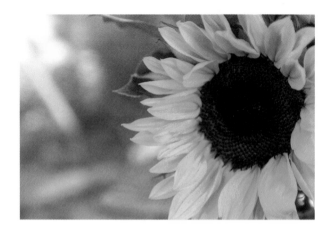

("teachers"), and according to Dr. Stanbury, the tribes there believe the "plant spirit enters the body and teaches us" (Plant Summit 2017). Plants have been shown to be sentient: they feel and respond accordingly to their environment, can anticipate possible responses, and act accordingly. Thus, the life of a plant will directly impact, scientifically and metaphysically, the essential oil it produces.

Beyond the scientific community, many cultures have long looked to plants for their attributes to maintain good health in humans. Plant medicine and the plant world are given an equal place among earth dwellers who acknowledge the intelligence and nourishment they provide to our air and body. Plants can do even more: along with developing defense mechanisms—e.g., thicker leaves, waxy coatings, spines, and thorns—against insects and herbivores, some have evolved to stave off certain predators through chemical messaging. What is fascinating about this type of communication is, not only does the individual single plant benefit, but there appear to be group benefits to neighboring plants and other creatures as well. For example, corn plants have been documented as releasing a volatile chemical substance into the air when a certain caterpillar begins to eat them. Unchecked, this caterpillar, the stem borer, can kill a corn plant. However, the plants have the ability to signal—to another species—the presence of the borer. A very specific enemy of the caterpillar arrives, a small wasp that lays its eggs in the caterpillar, providing relief to the corn plant and sustainability to the wasp.

who have had herbal or gardening experience or are food conscious are familiar with the overlapping link of plant health and our food sources. But did you know that trees and plants have been acknowledged by the scientific community as having cognition? Jill Stanbury, PhD, who specializes in herbal and natural medicine as well as leads ethnobotany field courses in the Amazon, shares that scientists have been able to document specific patterns produced by certain stimuli, or triggers, that create exacting results. These trigger-to-response patterns exhibit direct cognitive criteria of awareness and self-organizing. Although many scientists, says Dr. Stanbury, are unwilling to word it as such, they have adopted "minimal cognition" as the official acknowledgment. While plants do not possess the same organs and functions as the animal kingdom, they have electrical transmitters that communicate with their plant neighbors and other life forms, including humans. In the Amazon, plants are called *maestras*

Using nature's innate design lessens the use of chemical pesticides on your food and flowers. Farmers long have used the concept of companion planting, a unique combination of placing one plant near another to naturally prevent predators. For instance, marigolds, also known as calendula, when planted near all garden crops, stimulate vegetable growth and deter pests.

## WHY DO PLANTS CREATE ESSENTIAL OILS?

Plants have various levels of defense, including physical structure, color, and chemical substances. Plants do not need essential oils to be a plant. Not all plants have essential oils. Only a small group within a very large kingdom of plants are aromatic, approximately 10%. Primary metabolites are the most important structural components of a plant. These include amino acids, carbohydrates, lipids, and proteins as the building blocks of the plant. Secondary metabolites are the compounds that are synthesized by a plant and are limited in the plant kingdom to the family, genus, and species in which they appear. They are special. Because not every plant has essential oils, it is important to remember that they only come from certain plants that need to survive without the risk of overharvestation.

In the group of aromatic plants, essential oils are the secondary metabolites focused on here, but it is interesting to note that other secondary metabolites, such as tannins, are often studied in foods; for instance, wine and tea. Tannins are astringent and have a bitter flavor and are often desired in some cases. Essential oils, such as in geranium, cypress, and clary sage, can also have astringent qualities used topically.

Plants create essential oils for two primary reasons: protection and attraction. It is easy to connect the dots as to why a plant would produce chemical responses to insects, herbivores, fungus, bacteria, and other microbes. Sending signals to deter or ward off damaging attackers is a cry out for help and or a warning signal to stop. Some plants, according to Marcel Dicke, an entomologist from Wageningen University in the Netherlands, who along with biologist Maurice W. Sabelis at the University of Amsterdam, helped discover how plants communicate using volatiles, stated, "Some plants cry for help louder than others, some plants only whisper" (Richardson 2013).

Some plants produce secondary metabolites that are toxic to an attacker; other plants produce volatile vapors to attract natural predators. The "louder" the message that is "cried out" by a plant, the more natural predators and natural pollinators can find the plant.

The second reason essential oils are created is to attract. I would equate this to a plant's singing as opposed to the defensive shout-out. Bees are drawn by color and scent to plants that have pollen and nectar. Nectar contains sugars that provide carbohydrates as an energy source, and the pollen is used for its proteins and fats. Nectar is also what creates honey, hence honeys from different areas often have

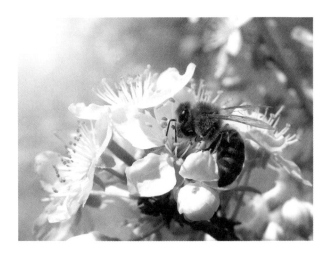

distinctive tastes due to the flowers from which the bees have collected nectar.

When bees and other insects make contact with a flowering plant, they help ensure cross-pollination, which furthers the plant species. In addition, animals that eat seeds and excrete them elsewhere also provide the plants with sustainability: the seeds are deposited in the ground along with built-in compost from the creature who ate it as a starter. The color of a plant and its blossom and scent are excellent signals to attract pollinators.

Have you ever been near a beautiful rose then moved as close as possible to smell its aroma? Or did you simply take a deep breath to gather the fragrance in the air? That single, deep breath immediately signals your parasympathetic nervous system to kick in. This is your "relax and rejuvenate" system. The scent of a rose draws you in, slows you down, and thus has a direct response on the mental and emotional parts

of you. Imagine the various scents flowers have on pollinators as they lure them to visit their blooms for pollen and nectar from miles away. For a plant that is stationary, it is a powerful device, a long-reaching summoning with lasting results.

## The Sun and the Moon

There is a circadian rhythm of the plant world, signaled by the sun and the moon, just as the human body responds to those celestial bodies.

When a plant germinates and the seed begins its journey to full-size plant, tree, or grass, it must have sunlight. The solar energy that warms the soil, enticing the leaves to reach upward toward the sky in spring, nourishes the plant with solar photons, encourages growth, and stimulates movement. Sometimes, these solar beams are too strong for some plants and so they grow in dappled or shaded areas. Other plants embrace heavy doses of sun, always giving me the impression of someone who stands face up to the sky to drink in the beams. Plants often adapt this sunshine to their advantage.

Bees are attracted to sweet smells, such as lemon scents. As a matter of fact, beekeepers who want to attract bees to their hives have found lemongrass essential oil to be an effective calling card to the new residence.

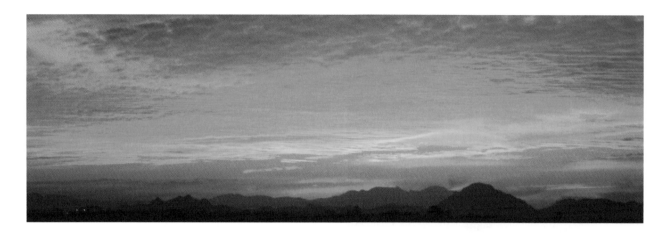

Think of what basking in the sun means to you. What words come to mind? *Happy, sunny, bright,* and *warm* are some of the properties of the sun's energy. These are properties of certain essential oils that also have an affinity with the sun. Imagine the bright, sunny disposition of citrus fruit, which need full sun to grow. These attributes can also have similar actions on our mind, emotions, body, and spiritual well-being: citrus aromas have the ability to lighten our moods, especially when life or thoughts feel heavy. The sun is transferred to your body, mind, and spirit through the citrus, which has absorbed its photons and is sharing them with you! David Crow succinctly imparts these thoughts: "The most important element in herbal medicine is sunlight. Sunlight comes to the earth and it is gathered using the green hands of the plants" (2016).

The moon is also a form of light energy, even though it is often associated with the darkness of night. The moon can be bright enough for us to see by, and often farmers plant seeds and harvest plants (and their essential oils!) according to the cycle of the moon. The harvest moon in autumn is special because it rises for three nights in a row around the time of sunset. All the other days of the year,

Just as essential oils have protective and attractive purposes in a plant, so can certain aromas have different effects on the physical body, mental functioning, and emotional well-being of a person. The scent from a single drop of citrus or rosemary oil can rejuvenate and stimulate the mind and awaken the senses. Others, such as lavender, rose, and neroli, are known for their relaxant properties. And still others, such as lavender, lemongrass, and some evergreens, trigger the immune system to respond to pathogens in the same way a plant would react to an invader.

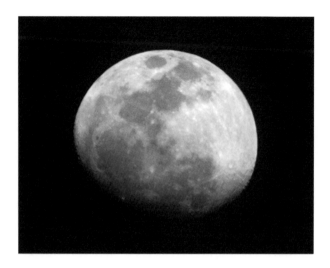

the moon's cyclical nature causes it to rise approximately 50 minutes later each night. Having the moon in the sky longer than usual during this time of a harvest moon means farmers can harvest well into the night, due to the extra light in the sky. This also means that any night the moon shines brightly, such as during a full moon, plants absorb higher amounts of the cooling lunar photons. On nights in which the moon is waning or waxing or "silent" as during a new moon, leaving the sky with less lunar light, plants absorb less lunar photons.

What does this matter to plants? Some plants actually bloom at night, not during the day. For them the moon embodies cool, soothing, soft energy, which is reflected in many of the softer magical aphrodisiacs and essential oils associated with soothing and quieting the mind and emotions, such as night-blooming jasmine (Crow 2014). Interestingly, the leaves of this plant, plucked by touch, are chosen individually with the knowledge that they will open that very night to impart their essential oils into the air. In a closed scent house, green tea leaves are laid out alongside or mixed with the blossoms for four hours, to absorb the intoxicating jasmine essential oils that become chemically bonded to create jasmine green tea. This process has been used for 1,000 years.

David Crow was taught by Dante Bolcato, an Italian psychotherapist and ethnobotanist who lives in Ecuador, about the qualities of the moon cycle when harvesting palo santo, a wonderful tree oil that has an unusual collection process. The tree must live a full life and die a natural death, and then when oil is extracted from the dead tree, the amount can vary depending on the moon cycle. Bolcato has observed harvesting through the full cycle from new to full moon and back yields a fuller complexity of palo santo essential oil.

## Earth and Sky

Soil and rain are the basic nutrient providers for plants, beyond the sun and carbon dioxide used for photosynthesis. They provide support, and if there is poor soil or depleted or excess water, a plant either has to learn to adapt or it can suffer.

One of the most telling aspects of an essential oil is where it grows in its native environment. Plants and trees all have adaptive qualities that are specific to the area in which they best thrive. For

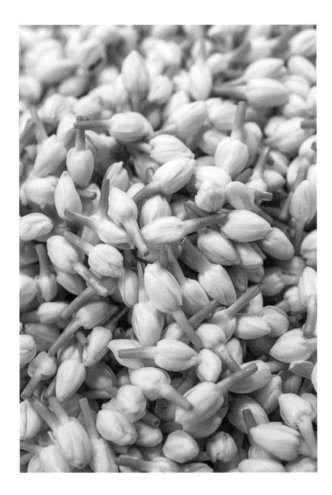

protected by spines or hard bark and shaded by small leaves, have to look as attractive as possible to a passing creature in the desert to ensure seed distribution. In the high deserts, such as in northern Nevada, the plants grow very close to the earth, mostly due to the dry winds, rarely rising upward unless they are a tree on a riverbank or natural spring, using water as a source of sustainability in a dry environment.

In the tropics, where water content is high in plants and trees, providing both physical and atmospheric support, leaves are wider and broader, and flowers have the luxury of display to match the size of the leaf. These flowers can give off strong scents far reaching in the wet climate to attract creatures and pollinators in the many layers of multiple tree canopies. Plants in general release a small amount of water into the air, and with many plants, there will be an increase in humidity. Fungi and bacteria, also abundant in wet climates, help break down all

instance, some desert plants have low-water-content foliage and develop other water-controlling characteristics. The lower the water content, the higher the oil potency, due to the lack of a dilutant in the structure. In the southwestern United States and in desert areas, cacti, small-leafed shrubs, and hardy desert trees are common. Seed pods and fruit, often

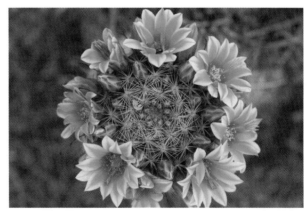

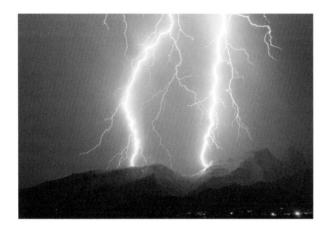

the foliage, but healthy plants need protection from premature decay. The essential oils produced can reflect the antimicrobial, antibacterial, and antifungal needs of such plants.

In semiarid and/or cooler locations affected by ether or air content, such as mountainous atmospheres, plants and trees have adaptive qualities unique to this environment. The higher up a mountain, the less oxygen is available. Plants and trees that survive, especially those that thrive in the atmosphere of less oxygen, have distinctive properties very different from those in the oxygen-rich tropics. They must transport their chemicals, proteins, and amino acids in different ways, which will change how an essential oil is used to provide maximum protection and attraction.

Each area has unique rain patterns. Some get consistent rain; others, very little. During monsoon rains in desert areas, the amount of rain goes from 0 to 100%, flooding dry riverbanks in a short period of time. Conversely, tropical areas have the ability to create higher moisture contents in the air and soil, and oftentimes nearby oceans or rivers serve as extra sources of water.

Heat also affects a plant's oil. Plants that are closer to the equator, such as Ecuador's palo santo, live in an environment that is warm all year round. These locations can be either tropical or desert but still receive direct sun for more days of the year than in other places of the world. Hot climates or hot weather can translate to essential oils' demonstrating warm physiological, emotional, digestive, or spiritual properties. Cooler temperatures or cooler atmospheres will produce essential oils that contain cooler wisdom. You might find that the more you

According to essential oil expert David Crow, warming and hot spices and herbs, such as cinnamon, basil, oregano, and thyme, are actually best used in their plant form. While their essential oils are available, these oils' concentration of chemical compounds is so strong that they can be damaging to skin and mucous membranes. To be safe, instead use the actual aromatic plant in cooking or teas. This is a wonderful way to get the benefit of a "hot" plant without the risk of a reaction or stress on the body. Many cultures and practices, such as Traditional Chinese Medicine and Ayurveda, have long recognized the value of using "hot" herbs and spices in their plant form (Crow 2016).

play with essential oils, the easier it will be to pick up on warming or cooling attributes.

## Time of Day

Some plants have bursts of energy to produce higher volumes of higher-potency oil at different times of day—and night! Flowers do not last a long time and therefore must be plucked when their oil is the highest, before the plant reclaims the energy needed to produce the bloom and drops its petals. Roses are best picked before dawn in the spring for the most fragrant oils; orange blossom (neroli), at high noon. Night-blooming jasmine is best picked when it blooms at midnight. In some species of oregano, reports David Crow, the constituent of carvacrol is higher at 10 a.m., but the same plant's thymol is higher at midnight. This is not the case for all plants; some respond to the amount of sunlight they receive without being tied to the solar/lunar clock. Clearly plants have an intelligence that adjusts to specific and individual protective and attractive needs.

## Humans Are Nature, Too

Humans share with plants the natural life cycle of birth, growth, peak energy, reproduction, decay, and death. Sometimes, it can appear we are moving through cycles similar to seasons. When snow

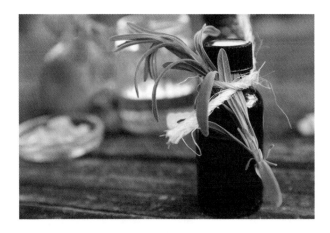

is on the ground, we may fail to realize how much energy is being circulated in the root system of plants and trees. But leaves on a tree have to come from somewhere, and the energy it takes to create a springtime blossom is a result of the life energy the tree sustained throughout winter. Similarly, there are occasions where we are processing thoughts and dreams deep within, but not showing anything on the outside . . . at least, not yet! When we are ready, we "spring" into action, our inspirations moving to the next stage of development: breaking ground and growing. Summer is when we are at our most experiential, reaching our peak adult potential, creating our own offspring, a maturity of life moving toward harvest: in autumn, we slow down, look back, gather what is important, and begin to release what no longer applies. In the later years of life, we pare down and let go of material items and create a simpler life, such is the time enjoyed after retirement. Similarly, in the fall, trees

Just as indigenous peoples from around the world ascribe sacredness to the power of plants and animals, acknowledging a connection between species is a valuable learning and teaching experience. Follow their lead and open all of your senses to the magic of essential oils.

"If we're only listening for words—for language in human terms—then we're barely listening at all! The world speaks to us in the ancient tongue of touch and color, texture and fragrance, through taste and breath and every part of our senses." —Kiva Rose

Plants pull their energy away from the periphery when they are depleted, much as a body will direct energy toward organs and away from extremities if distressed. It is nature's response to support the most vital components that keep the functioning unit alive. Some plants "rest" by folding their flowers inward at sunset, often by spiraling them closed, similar to humans' curling up to sleep at night.

Reminders of how connected humans are to nature will be one of the most important lessons a novice to essential oils can experience and it will most certainly deepen the understanding of those who have greater familiarity.

release their leaves so as to gather energy for the root system to sustain them during winter, and so as people release their human body in winter, the cycle begins again with a new generation in the springtime of life.

Parallels between humans and nature allow a synergistic sharing on planet Earth. As plants give us oxygen and we, in return, give them carbon dioxide, there are other biocompatible components we share with each other. Essential oils are part of plants, but are incredibly concentrated. Just as too much food and drink is often taxing on a body and sometimes harmful, these oils are more biocompatible when diluted (see Chapter 5).

Scientifically speaking, the human body and the plant kingdom have parallels in transmitters of electrical currents to relay needs for sustainability.

## Doctrine of Signatures

The Doctrine of Signatures (DOS) is not considered a true scientific form of analysis. However, its use of observation of color, shape, taste, and habitat in which a plant grows, and sometimes, the plant's stages of development, demonstrates the connection between humans and the natural world. Folkloric applications of plants have withstood hundreds, if not thousands, of years. These relationships go much deeper for master herbalists, who gain a lot from the language of identifying markers in plant expressions. The DOS matches how a plant looks to its potential healing powers within the human body, specifically which organs it can assist. Certainly the history of using the DOS goes back before science could confirm many of the amazing nutritive values in these applications, such as vitamins.

Paracelsus (1493–1541), an alchemist from the time of the Renaissance, coined the term "Doctrine of Signatures," but its concept goes back farther in recorded history, to Greek botanist Dioscorides (AD 40–90). However, the idea of using the "signature of all things," as Jacob Boehme titled his book on the subject (1621), helped expand the uses and natural descriptions of the DOS.

Certainly, poets and philosophers have gathered much from the observation of plants. Many early alchemists used astrology to assign certain relationships of plants to planets. Poet Johann von Goethe (1749–1832) broke away from this by thinking of the plant more in terms of "its relationship to the sun, heights and the elements of fire and air," writes herbalist Matthew Wood, who goes on to say that philosopher and scientist Rudolf Steiner further invited the uses of observation to include "perception (physical observation), feeling, thinking, and intuition. The use of intuition promotes observation as a whole, rather than in pieces." What we can glean from this philosophy, when learning about essential oils, is that there is more than meets the eye. This sings a similar tune to the holistic approach of Marguerite Maury.

The Doctrine of Signatures looks for the following kinds of characteristics (this is a simplified list):

- *Color:* Green for nourishment and blood cleansing (nettle); yellow equates to bile and digestion (dandelion); red, to heat-related items and is used for cooling (red clover); blue or purple for blood purification (echinacea); black for tissue death (black cohosh); white for bone healing (white roots of comfrey)
- *Shape:* Long, tubular shapes for urinary tract support; kidney-shape bean pods for kidneys; walnuts for brain
- *Habitat:* Wet habitats for diseases of wetness (lungs, colds) or by clear water (diuretic)

Examples of signatures:

- *Beets:* The deep red-purple color of blood closely resembles the juice and body of a beet. Beets help clean the blood and may assist in lowering blood pressure.
- *Carrots:* When sliced crosswise, carrots mirror the human eye. Science has been able to prove

### MYTH: ESSENTIAL OILS ARE THE LIFE BLOOD OF THE PLANT.

This is not true. If it were, every plant would contain essential oils. But only a small percentage of the entire plant kingdom produces them. Dr. Robert Pappas says that essential oils act more like sweat in the human body than they do any other body fluid.

the carotenoids in carrots support human eye health.

- *Tomatoes:* The four sections of the inner tomato closely resemble the four chambers of the heart. Tomatoes' lycopene is known to support cardio-vascular health.
- *Walnuts:* Contained in a hard shell, this oddly wrinkled nut has two symmetrical halves that closely resemble the human brain: two fleshy hemispheres within a protective skull. Walnuts contain vitamin E, which may assist in brain health and cognitive disorders.

## How Plants Express Themselves

There is a basic biology to all living organisms. Certain identifying properties distinguish a plant from a mammal as well as from other creatures. In a fashion similar to the Doctrine of Signatures, observation of how plants express themselves can be helpful in remembering certain properties of an essential oil. Imagine this as *partial* qualities expressed in a personality. Partial, because all the other attributes of the plant will also go into the personality, such as whether it is a sun- or moon-loving plant. Here are a few ways to remember the expressions of plants that you will meet in Part 3 of this book.

- *Seeds (and nuts)* hold the matrix, or blueprint, of the entire plant; they are its wisdom and deepest inner nature. Their job is to go out into the world, discover new experiences, and perpetuate the species. Seeds are pure potential and can help find the potential within and express it outwardly.
- *Stems* support reaching out and letting go with the assistance of an internal anchor. It's okay to move forward.
- *Leaves and needles* signify opening, expanding, inviting the breath of life to exchange in and out.
- *Flowers* denote love, creativity, freedom to be oneself, sensory, expressiveness, spontaneity, living in the moment.
- *Fruits* demonstrate fertility of intention, joyfulness, protection until it is no longer needed, sweetness and lightness in life.
- *Woods* provide stability, anchored motion, support, encouraging compassion through longevity, slowing down.
- *Resins* have self-healing properties, healing the inner wounds of experience, bringing inspira-

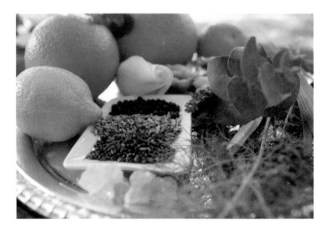

tion forward from the unseen, seeing within, protection, unwavering strength and flexibility.
- *Roots and rhizomes* supply groundedness, deep resources, warmth, encouragement.

## Where Plants Store Essential Oils

Essential oils contain antibacterial, antimicrobial, and antiviral properties to protect their parent plant. This can translate to the value of what these oils can do for humans, once we understand how they work in their own natural environment.

Pine and cypress, for instance, produce an oil that safeguards the trees' well-being. This chemical signaling blankets the entire area in a forest, communicating with other trees to produce a collaborative atmospheric shift, keeping the forests cool and maintaining a certain level of humidity in the air. In other words, it signals the forest to breathe. Interestingly enough, when most people smell the scent of these trees in nature, they take a deeper breath. Essential oils from the forest trees are often used for their antimicrobial power to support lung and sinus health.

It is very easy to smell the fragrance of most flowers just by being near them. Some plants carry essential oils very close to the surface—so close that the tiny tarsus (foot) of an insect is enough to release their vapors into the air. Other plants require being slightly disturbed or gently bruised to release their oils. And certain oils are released only when there is distinct disturbance, such as cutting its root.

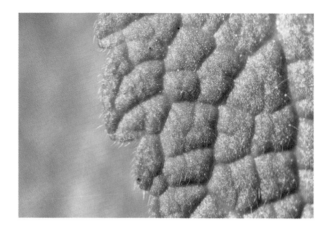

The chemical compounds in citrus help keep pests away as it grows and ripens. As the fruit matures, the same chemical component assists in breaking down the thick rind so creatures can eat the fruit and spread the seeds. In human application, citrus has been found to bring out calmer and sunnier dispositions, protecting when needed and then showing that life can be light and juicy!

Essential oils are found either outside or inside a plant's structure. External secretory structures or cells, called glandular trichomes, are easily "burst" to release the essential oils. They act as both protectors and attractants to the plant. Plants with glandular trichomes that contain essential oils include lavender, basil, marjoram, rosemary, oregano, melissa (a.k.a. lemon balm), and spearmint.

Internal secretory structures are classified as either cavities or ducts, depending on the plant and purpose. They are held between cells and released when disturbed or when the neighboring cell is dam-

Essential oils are found in different places within an aromatic plant. You will find the more you learn about which part of the plant an essential oil is derived from, the more you learn about the plant itself and the oil's personality and purpose. Many plants, such as geranium, have essential oils in their leaves; lavender, in its flowers. Outer layers of rinds in citrus, as in sweet orange and lemon, are another place where essential oils are found. Others oils, such as palo santo and cinnamon, are in stems, twigs, branches, or bark. Seeds and nuts also contain precious oils, as does the root system of ginger and vetiver. Each plant stores and uses the essential oils differently. Resin is a thick, viscous fluid that seals wounds in a tree, and in the aromatic plant family also contains essential oils, as in the case of frankincense and myrrh. Grasses, such as lemongrass, also contain essential oils.

contains secretory cells and its spicy, warm scent is really only released once the root has been cut. That is, when intact, ginger does not release any distinguishable aroma. Other examples of plants with secretory cells are black pepper and nutmeg.

All plants have stomata, pores that open when exposed to light, allowing a gaseous exchange called transpiration: when water vapors (which contain oxygen) exit the plant into the air and carbon dioxide enter into the plant. That carbon dioxide is necessary for photosynthesis, which is how plants create food and oxygen. According to the Plant and Soil Sciences Library, stomata are triggered by light, and they are most sensitive to the blue light of sunrise. It is almost as if the plant wakes up and takes a deep breath to greet the day just as the sun appears. (Note: Transpiration is the respiration process common to all plants, not the release of essential oils by a select few.)

aged or disintegrates. Secretory cavities are found in clove buds and eucalyptus; citruses, such as lemon and orange; and resins from frankincense and myrrh trees. Ducts are more elongated than cavities and are found in Roman and German chamomiles, fir, cedar, spruce, and pine, as well as in fennel and carrot seeds.

Secretory cells are very different from external glands or internal cavities or ducts. The oils held in these cells are released only with a specific disturbance to the plant. Ginger, a fibrous rhizome,

## Harvesting and Processing

The closest to the natural world of a plant that you can get, the better. This means wild harvested (often by hand in the natural terrain of the plant), organic (no pesticides, no artificial additives to the soil or water, and no chemical sprays), and sustainably supported (not depleting the land nor the plant's longevity on the planet).

Cultivated crops, simply put, are farms. There is nothing wrong with farms, especially when a crop is supported by good, nutritious soil and plenty of clean water and is harvested with care. Farming on depleted soils with impure water or spraying with chemical pesticides, on the other hand, will create a crop that reflects the poor environment in which it was grown. Whenever possible, avoid chemically sprayed crops, as those chemicals can get into the essential oils. Essential oils are concentrated. The last thing you want is a concentration of added poison.

When scientists have figured out the chemistry of a particular desired attribute, they may synthetically produce it in a lab and then use the result in a product. But you may find the broad, synergetic properties of a real plant produce a better, lasting effect than does a singled-out component. In other words, sometimes a single component is not as powerful on its own. Other times, a single component is what makes (or breaks) a product. For instance, lavender chemical "fragrances" created by adding linalool are no match for those that contain genuine lavender essential oil.

## DISTILLATION AND OTHER EXTRACTIONS

Steam distillation, hydrodistillation, codistillation, maceration, and expression are the different ways essential oils are gathered from a plant. In addition, solvents may be employed if working with especially delicate botanicals.

*Distillation* uses a still to release the volatile components, the essential oils. Hot steam rising from a mixture of water and plant material moves into a long tube and begins to fill it to the point

> ### MYTH: ESSENTIAL OILS ARE NATURAL, SAFE, AND CAN BE USED FREELY.
>
> Anyone who has had any exposure to the natural elements of nature knows that they are powerful. Wind can be a welcome breeze or knock a town flat in a tornado. Water can be a source of life or wash away an entire coastline in a tsunami. Respecting the power of nature is superimportant. Calling something a "natural" product does not mean thoughtless usage is safe. Understanding the difference between "natural" and "harmless" can be totally different according to context. Respect the information about each individual oil and use it appropriately. Always dilute.

where it follows the length of the tubing. The tubing is then circled around a cooling bath. Once that hot steam meets the cooling bath, it once again forms a liquid, like a cloud making rain. When the liquid comes out of the tubing, it is captured in a separatory funnel where the water, called hydrolat or hydrosol, is allowed to accumulate. A natural separation of the oil and water occurs; the oil is what we call essential oils. The hydrolat and the essential oils are then separated into different containers, labeled, and made ready for storage, use, or sale.

The difference between water distillation, hydrodistillation, and codistillation is how the water and

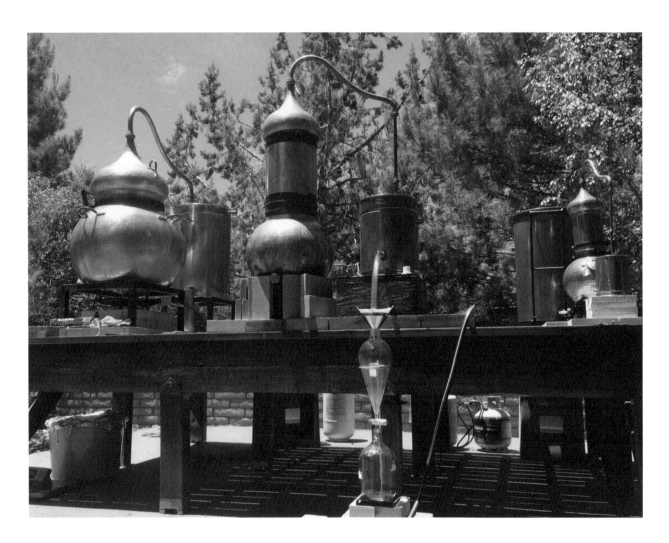

plant material, called the charge, are placed within the still. *Water distillation* places water *below* the charge, which is placed above the water on a metal grate, and is distilled. *Hydrodistillation* uses the charge *in* the water at the bottom of the still, much like making soup. *Codistillation* uses the plant charge both *in* the big still compartment and *above* in the "hat" of the still. *Steam distillation* takes place when steam is injected into the still.

*Expression* usually applies to citrus, due to

essential oils' being in the rind. Think of the fresh aroma created by peeling an orange—citrus rind needs to be disturbed to break it open and release its oils. This process was once called cold pressing, as originally it was done by using a cold sponge to press the fruit that had been soaked in warm water to open the rind. Afterward, the water and juice were removed, and then the oil syphoned off.

*Maceration* is used to release essential oils in warm water by reducing the enzymes binding the essential oils in plants such as onion, garlic, wintergreen, and bitter almond.

Other methods of obtaining essential oils are percolation, enfleurage, solvent extraction, absolutes, and $CO_2$ supercritical extraction:

*Percolation* happens when steam is brought in from the top of the still, rather than from the bottom.

*Enfleurage* uses the high absorbency rate of animal fats to soak in the essential oils from a plant, especially those that continue to emanate their aromatic vapors after harvest, such as jasmine. It is rare to find this in the world of aromatherapy, due to expense. It is considered more of a historic method in the Grasse region of France, but it is still used there.

*Solvent extraction* uses solvents to pull out the chlorophyll and other plant tissue to move it out of the way to gain access to the essential oils. This method is used for delicate petals of flowers that are too sensitive to go through a distillation process. It is the first phase in creating an absolute.

*Absolutes* are when the solvent extraction, which

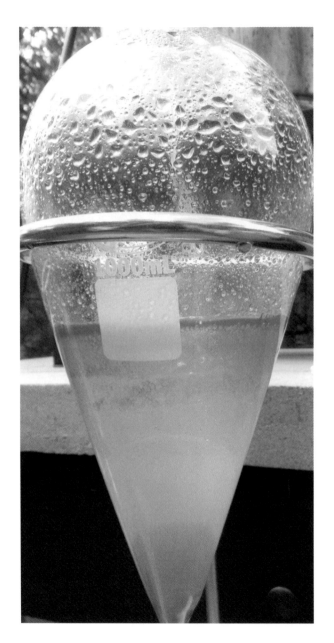

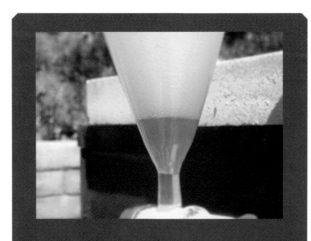

Almost all essential oils rise to the top of water. However, there are some exceptions to this rule. Clove bud is much denser than water and sinks at the end of the distillation process. The warm aroma that accompanies the clove bud while it distilled reminded me of fresh, out-of-the-oven banana bread or bananas foster! As an essential oil, though, it has the distinctive smell associated with cloves. Always be open to interesting moments that essential oils can teach you!

is thick and viscous, is diluted with alcohol to make it a bit more fluid and more user-friendly. Absolutes are often used for subtle therapies, such as psychological support, due to their highly aromatic concentrations. The thinner the absolute, the lesser the grade (that means it has more alcohol).

As for *CO$_2$ supercritical extractions*, carbon dioxide (CO$_2$) is used to force the volatile vapors out of a charge under tightly controlled, very specific pressure and temperatures (think pressure cooker). As no water is used in the process while the CO$_2$ extracts the oils, the end result is essential oils that have not been damaged by steam heat. This also means no hydrosol is created, as occurs in steam distillation. Because of the controlled environments with this process, aromas and overall chemistry are closer to the actual botanical aroma and taste (some are used in the food and beverage industry for flavoring). This is a widely expanding offshoot of traditional aromatherapy.

*Hydrolat* is a French term, from *hydro* ("water") and *lait* ("milk"), for the milky white substance often produced when first distilled. *Hydrosol*, coined in the United States by Ann Harmon, is also an accepted term for the distilled waters, describing the suspended state: hydro + sol(ution). Most historians, perfumers, and nonprofessionals called this *flower water*, because it retained a softer version of the flowery scent of the original plant. Flower waters were used long before the advent of distilling essential oils, for cooking, drinking, and fragrance. Now we know they are more biocompatible than essential oils, due to their low essential oil and high water ratio. Today, hydrosols are used as facial toners, in place of regular water in diffusers, compresses, mouthwashes, and room fresheners. They are especially nice to use with children.

There is some controversy among aromatherapists as to whether some carbon dioxides remain in the essential oil. So far, all testing has shown that the residual amount is so minute as to be of no concern, but purists of the traditional methods tend to be partial to distilled oils. Some argue that pesticides from conventionally grown plants may carry over through the $CO_2$ supercritical extraction process. Therefore, it is ideal to use organic plant resources to ensure an unadulterated $CO_2$ extract. There are benefits to all methods of obtaining essential oils.

$CO_2$ extractions can have different qualities than those produced by steam. Frankincense, for instance, exhibits more immunity-enhancing components and anti-inflammatory activity in a $CO_2$ extraction than it does when distilled. $CO_2$ extractions also tend to have a different, sometimes stronger, aroma.

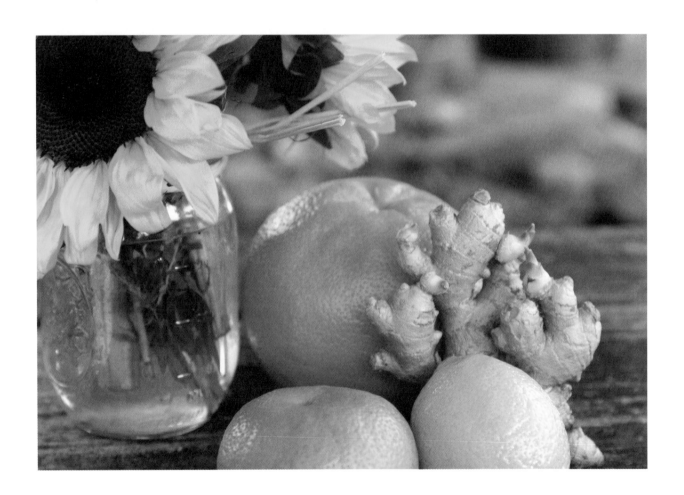

# CHAPTER 3

# Proper Names: Latin Binomials and Chemical Components

*Natura nihil facit frustra. (Nature does nothing in vain.)*
—Latin saying

## Latin Binomials and Special Titles

Meeting someone casually for the first time, I am often introduced by my first name only. However, for professional purposes, such as formal introductions at presentations, I am often introduced with my full name and a small biography.

The names of essential oils have a similar split. People are often casually introduced to an oil by its plant's common name, usually consisting of one or two words, such as lavender or clary sage. These work just fine as long as greater specificity is not necessary. But I am quickly reminded of fourth grade, when there were four Jennifers in my class. Distinguishing among them wasn't as easy as adding their surname's initial, because two had the same last initial. And so for the rest of their school years, they were known as Jenny, Jennie, Jennifer, and Jennifer H. Just as saying, "I know Jennifer!" may be quickly followed by "Which one?" There are more than 70 different species of lavender. That would be like having 70-plus Jennifers in the room when you need one specific Jennifer to do a job. Hence, more than just the common name may be needed to distinguish an essential oil.

Science has a wonderful way of grouping together items that share similarities:

*Taxonomy* was developed in the 1730s by Carolus Linnaeus as a way to classify animals, minerals, and plants.

*Nomenclature* is the naming of these items in a

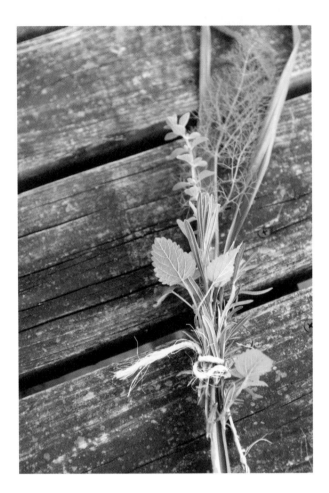

A plant's *Latin binomial*, also known as its botanical name, consists of the *genus* as its first name, which is always capitalized (think surname) and the *species*, its second name, always in lowercase (think given name). Both are written in italics. Some plants have alternative names in Latin, depending on who assigned the binomial to them.

A plant's *common name*, what most people call it (think nickname), is not italicized, and usually consists of one or two simple words. Sometimes a plant has more than one common name.

You probably won't use Latin binomials in everyday conversation. However, they will be helpful if you need to specify which plant you mean or want to check the label of a bottle of essential oil to ensure that it is the correct product for your purpose. Be sure to use the full binomial in such cases, as a genus may encompass numerous species, each with distinctive characteristics.

Botanical names are even more important as you travel the world. All plants have a Latin name, but common names may be different according to location and culture (e.g., in Spain, a name may be Jose; in America, Joseph, but the Latin for both is Josephus wherever you go). For this reason, Latin is used worldwide as the language of medicine and botany. Clinical aromatherapist, educator, and author Liz Fulcher shares a story from her Aromatic Wisdom podcast of a client of hers, traveling abroad, who was able to obtain clary sage essential oil despite a language barrier, by using its Latin botanical name, *Salvia sclarea*, to ask for it!

way that identifies them clearly through eight different levels. Four examples of this layered system are kingdom, family, genus (pl. genera), and species, all of which terms are in Latin.

*Families* categorize large groups within a specific kingdom, which helps identify certain similarities that only a particular family possesses.

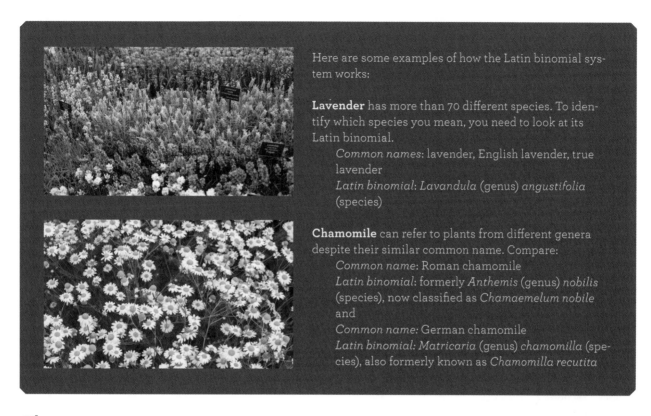

Here are some examples of how the Latin binomial system works:

**Lavender** has more than 70 different species. To identify which species you mean, you need to look at its Latin binomial.
> *Common names*: lavender, English lavender, true lavender
> *Latin binomial*: *Lavandula* (genus) *angustifolia* (species)

**Chamomile** can refer to plants from different genera despite their similar common name. Compare:
> *Common name*: Roman chamomile
> *Latin binomial*: formerly *Anthemis* (genus) *nobilis* (species), now classified as *Chamaemelum nobile*
> and
> *Common name:* German chamomile
> *Latin binomial: Matricaria* (genus) *chamomilla* (species), also formerly known as *Chamomilla recutita*

## Chemotypes

Twins, triplets, and the like usually fall into two categories: identical and fraternal. *Identical* means the fetuses split apart after conception, and so they are the same sex and share all the same physical qualities; although some subtle differences will allow you to tell them apart, these may not be immediately obvious. *Fraternal* means they were separate entities in the womb from the start; they look different, can be of different sexes, and are often mistaken for simply being siblings.

Taking this idea to the botanical world, shifts in the air, soil, water, nutrients, and other conditions, perhaps as simple as growing on the far side of the mountain away from the sea, may change a plant ever so slightly. It might look the same on the outside, but the chemicals inside are different.

When such a natural change has occurred, this is referred to as the plant's *chemotype*, abbreviated as "ct.," which follows the name of its plant species (without italics). Chemotypes are important when you are looking for a specific property within that

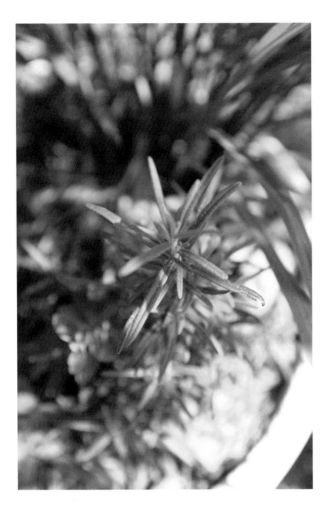

rosemary ct. verbenone, commonly shortened to "rosemary verbenone," is one of three rosemary chemotype "triplets" (not an aromatherapy technical term!); the others are *Rosmarinus officinalis* ct. 1,8 cineole, and *Rosmarinus officinalis* ct. camphor. All three belong to the same family, genus, and species, varying only by the respective heightened chemicals within the plant.

## Chemistry

Knowing the chemistry of essential oils is not necessary for the beginner, but it can help you understand why certain oils work better than others for particular uses.

Terpenes comprise the largest chemical group (more than 30,000 identified) in essential oils. Here are their primary classifications as related to aromatherapy:

**Monoterpenes:** Essential oils that contain monoterpenes do best stored in the refrigerator or in a cold room because they are prone to oxidation, which can lead to skin sensitivity. They evaporate very quickly, which means they can be drying to the body. These compounds do not mix with water (you will not find them in hydrosols). They are antimicrobial as well as really great for diffusers and creating an uplifting environment. These are often detected first in a blend as a top note (i.e., they evaporate into the air faster than other components). *Examples:* sweet

plant species. Often, the aroma is changed slightly due to the altered chemical composition, which can be helpful for beginners in learning which oil is which. Plus, there is usually a sharper variety and a softer variety, aromatically speaking.

*Rosmarinus officinalis* ct. verbenone, a.k.a.

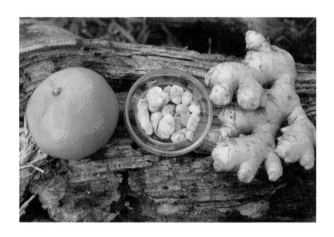

orange, lemon, Scot's pine, cypress. *Chemical compound examples:* d-limonene, α-pinene, terpinolene.

**Sesquiterpenes:** These evaporate a bit slower than monoterpenes, but also do not do well with water, so you won't find them in hydrosols, either. Because they are slightly heavier than monoterpenes, they oxidize a bit slower as well. These are often associated as middle notes in a blend because of their slightly slower volatile nature. These compounds have really great anti-inflammatory actions, along with antispasmodic and calming properties for the nervous system. *Examples:* ginger, helichrysum, clary sage, German chamomile. *Chemical compound examples:* chamazulene, ar-acurcumene, zingiberene.

**Monoterpene alcohols (a.k.a. monoterpenols):** These are monoterpenes with added alcohol chemicals. These smell nice and are generally useful for children and the elderly. They are often found in skin products, as they can tolerate some solubility in water. These compounds are good for those who need parasympathetic ("rest and rejuvenate") nervous system support. Known for being antifungal, antimicrobial, and antiviral as well as analgesic (pain relieving), anti-inflammatory, and calming. *Examples:* lavender, clary sage, sweet marjoram, geranium. *Chemical compound examples:* borneol, linalool, menthol.

**Sesquiterpene alcohols (a.k.a. sesquiterpenols):** These are sesquiterpenes with added alcohol. These tend to be a bit thicker (viscous) in feel than monoterpenols and are great to add to vegetable-based carrier oils. These are the helpers you will find in muscle-, nerve-, and lymph-supportive blends. They are also antifungal, anti-inflammatory, and antispasmodic, as well as sedative. You will definitely find these in skin-care recipes. *Examples:* helichrysum, German chamomile, sandalwood, patchouli. *Chemical compound examples:* a-bisabolol, α(alpha)- and β(beta)-santalol, patchoulol.

**Esters:** These are interesting because they occur only when an alcohol has had a reaction with an organic acid. They are analgesic, antibacterial, anti-inflammatory, cooling, and sedative. These compounds relieve tension in the body and the mind/emotion connection. *Examples:* Roman chamomile, clary sage, lavender, ylang-ylang. *Chemical compound examples:* bornyl acetate, methyl salicylate, terpineol acetate. *Caution:* Two special esters you

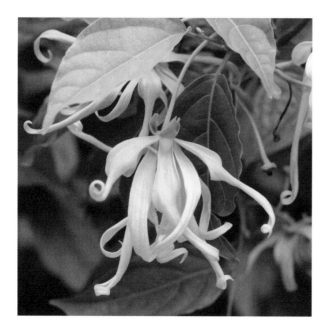

diffusers to help clear the air of bacteria. They are also antifungal, provide anti-inflammatory support, are sedative, and relieve anxiety. *Examples:* melissa (lemon balm), lemongrass, lemon eucalyptus, citronella. *Chemical compound examples:* citronellal, citral, geranial, neral.

**Ketones:** Essential oils that contain ketones are not prone to oxidization, which means they are more stable in the bottle and in a blend; consequently, you will find them in some hydrosols. They are strong agents against stuck mucus and can help with wound healing and reducing inflammation. An interesting fact: A unique ketone called nootkatone is solely responsible for the aroma of grapefruit! *Examples:* peppermint, rosemary, spearmint, thyme ct. camphor. *Chemical compound examples:* camphor, menthone, thujone. *Caution:* Do not use the following during pregnancy or breastfeeding: camphor, sage (*Salvia officinalis*), rue, mugwort, wormwood, thuja, or pennyroyal.

**Phenols:** *Caution:* Not only must essential oils that contain phenols be highly diluted in a carrier oil, but they should also not be used for extended periods of time—they can be too much for the liver to process. They can also be damaging to the skin if not handled with care. When used properly, they are strongly antibacterial (one of the best) as well as fantastically antifungal. They are warming (some consider these "hot" oils), and can enhance the immune, digestive, and respiratory systems—if used with

may have heard of, birch and wintergreen, must not be used with children, pregnant or nursing women, anyone with damaged skin, or anyone who is taking blood thinners. These two esters contain a naturally occurring aspirin-like compound, which means that both can act as blood thinners. As a general comparison for safety purposes, one teaspoon of either of those oils is similar to 21 adult aspirins.

**Aldehydes:** Compounds that contain aldehydes must always be diluted in a carrier, due to their high potential for skin irritation. Aldehydes often have a slightly fruity aroma, which might remind you to definitely dilute. They are wonderful antivirals and you will often find them in cleaning products or

care. Diffusers are best for an airborne or respiratory antimicrobial purpose. *Examples:* basil, thyme, oregano, winter savory. *Chemical compound examples:* carvacrol, thymol, eugenol (also classified as a phenylpropanoid). *Caution:* Some phenols can present some potential dangers for pregnant and breastfeeding women.

**Phenylpropanoids:** That warm, spicy scent in cinnamon and clove is from the components of this category. Their actions are very pronounced when in an essential oil. According to master herbalist and aromatherapist Jade Shutes, these compounds "are strengthening, yet stimulating to the nervous system." They are anti-inflammatory and antimicrobial, great for airborne purification (use diffuser), and assist with digestion. *Examples:* anise, basil, cinnamon, clove, fennel. *Chemical compound examples:* cis-anethole (toxic), trans-anethole (found in fennel), eugenol. *Caution:* Use all phenylpropanoids in short-term, highly diluted blends only! Consult a doctor before using any phenylpropanoid and consult a qualified aromatherapist for additional essential oil safety information during pregnancy and breastfeeding. Avoid any use of fennel during pregnancy, breastfeeding, endometriosis, and estrogen-dependent cancers.

**Oxides:** These compounds definitely do not like air and oxygen. They are very light and will oxidize if exposed to heat. They are, however, wonderful analgesics and are superb for respiratory

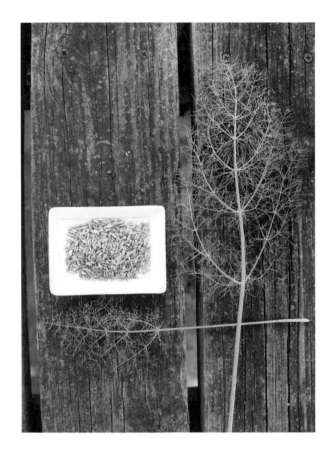

support. Besides being antiviral, they are also anti-inflammatory. Buy these in small containers, store properly, and use within a year. *Examples:* eucalyptus, tea tree, German chamomile, bay laurel. *Chemical compound examples:* 1,8 cineole (a.k.a. eucalyptol), rose oxide, sclareol.

**Sesquiterpene lactones:** These are fairly neutral compounds that are neither warming nor cooling per se, and even though more than 3,000 lactones have been identified, they are not readily found in many essential oils. They are, however, extremely effective with mucus issues, such as asthma and bronchitis. They are also antibacterial and antifungal. *Examples:* inula, catnip. *Chemical compound examples:* alantolactone, isolantolactone, neptalacton.

**Furanocoumarins:** *Caution:* These compounds create photosensitivity (meaning you will burn very badly in the sun or on a tanning bed and not know it until it is too late). They are best in highly diluted blends, especially if used for topical applications on your skin. *Wait at least 12 to 24 hours before sun or UV exposure.* This is a serious recommendation; even citrus juice contains these compounds and can potentially cause blisters and burns if not properly handled. On the plus side, they are antibacterial, anti-inflammatory, and antimicrobial. I like to think of these as nighttime oils, best used before bed or in the early evening for their relaxing properties. They can be used safely in rinse-off products, such as hand soap, due to their immediately being washed away, according to Tisserand and Young in their *Essential Oil Safety* guide, 2e (2012). *Examples:* bergamot, angelica root, and many citrus essential oils. *Chemical compound examples:* angelicin, bergapten.

## Assessing Essential Oils' Purity

Gas chromatography (GC) and mass spectrometry (MS) are two different tests used to determine the chemical constituent makeup of a particular essential oil.

*Gas chromatography* plots on a graph the volatile movement of each constituent by the speed and time it takes for the oil's vapors to go through the machine. If suspicious peaks show up outside the normal range of constituent fluctuations, such markers are noted as possible adulterations.

*Mass spectrometry* is the process whereby chemical compounds are identified by the ion mass unique to each constituent.

GC/MS findings are helpful in identifying pure essential oils; that is, oils that are free from contaminates. They keep essential oil distillers, distributors, and retail companies a bit more honest. A test that indicates an adulterated result means the oil is not safe to use therapeutically. However, these tests do not distinguish the quality of an essential oil or whether it works therapeutically. They are only a baseline of chemical identification and adulteration markers. Aromatherapist Joy Muscchio says fizzy and flat champagne will test the same chemically, but the value is definitely different! The same happens with relying solely on test results; it lacks the vitality of the oil.

Essential oils are distilled in batches. Not all

essential oil bottles list the batch number, but it can be helpful in following up if there is ever a problem. But do not be fooled into thinking that just because a batch number is supplied, that product is pure. Dr. Robert Pappas, an independent essential oils chemist who performs GC/MS testing for companies, has exposed several companies that have sold adulterated essential oils with batch numbers on the packaging. They can create a false sense of authenticity.

Many companies are moving toward using GC/MS reports to prove their products' purity. The only way to know the purity of an essential oil is to test a sample of every new batch a company purchases (and sells). Each test provides validity for that individual batch only; a company that purchased essential oils from a distiller cannot use those results for future batches. Testing takes time and is expensive if you are doing a lot of testing. As a result, not every reputable company tests its oils, or every batch. Factors that may affect the test results include the relationship the company has with its distiller or whether the company itself distills its oils, and how many hands an oil passes through before it reaches the firm. Sometimes things happen that are beyond a company's control, hence testing is becoming more predominate, and some even say, necessary. One also must consider that several major distilleries around the world distribute their oils worldwide, and the majority of distributors probably have some crossover in their product purchasing; that is, certain essential oils likely come from the same few distilleries.

A low price may indicate that essential oils might not pass a GC/MS report. In general, shop wisely: your local convenience or bargain store is not the place to get high-quality essential oils.

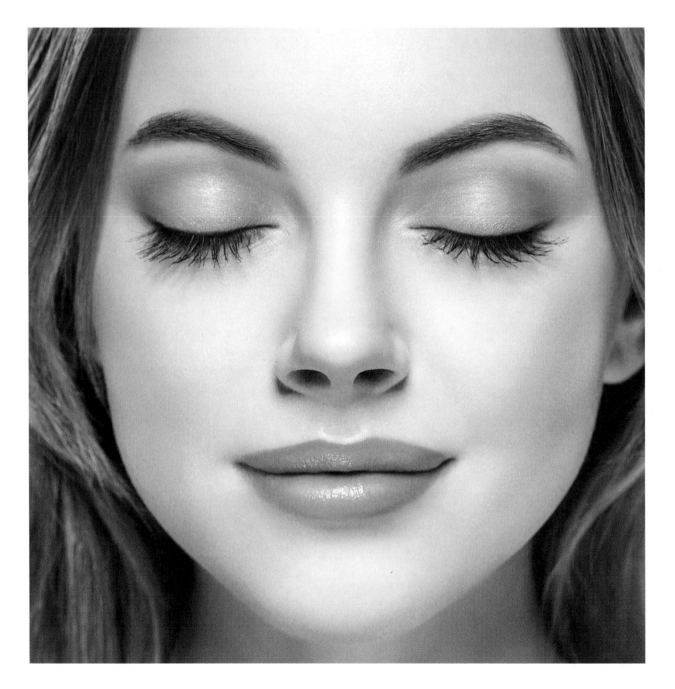

# CHAPTER 4

# Being Human

*One of the first conditions of happiness is that the link between Man and Nature shall not be broken.* —Leo Tolstoy

There are many sides to being human, but it is quite interesting to note that some of our longest known and most widely used philosophies concern our relationship with nature. These include:

*The Five Element Theory of Traditional Chinese Medicine* conveys how we express our complexity and individuality via physical, emotional, mental, and spiritual tendencies, challenges, and auspicious attributes. This system uses the physical elements of water, wood, fire, earth, and metal, which can be simplified in a life cycle as birth, growth, expression, togetherness, and letting go.

*The Indian system of Ayurveda*, which predates the Five Element Theory, describes human nature according to three *doshas*: Vata, Pitta, and Kapha, which describe different combinations of five natural elements: ether, air, fire, earth, and water.

*The Four Humors*, the youngest of these philos- ophies, dating back to ancient Greek medicine, describe the four physical metabolic processes— *sanguine*, *phlegmatic*, *choleric*, and *melancholic*, respectively—that occur within the four natural elements of air, water, fire, and earth.

Each of these philosophies attempts to connect with and understand the natural world's patterns and the human condition. None is rooted in a particular exclusive religion.

Essential oils can be described as providing humans with different (sometimes overlapping) effects: physical, emotional, mental, and spiritual. Knowing how the human system works can help you identify the best essential oil to support whichever system needs assistance.

Let's take a brief look at the many facets of being human and their relationship with essential oils.

# Breathing

## THE RESPIRATORY SYSTEM

In the study of Jin Shin Jyutsu, a physio-philosophy of the art of harmonizing the life force within the body, breathing is described as the giving and receiving of life. There is no "taking" a breath; rather, it is an exchange from the internal alchemy of the body to the external alchemy of the world in which it lives. Human respiration does not require light to take place, whereas for a plant, light *is* necessary to trigger the exchange properly (photosynthesis depends on light). Although humans do not have to think about breathing, breathing with consciousness creates an awareness that is very beneficial when using essential oils. There is something quite satisfying in a deep breath's effecting a complete release of any tension in the body and in the mind. It is like hitting reset.

The respiratory system, which supplies oxygen to the body while expelling carbon dioxide, is symbiotic with a plant's cycle of respiration and transpiration. The scents of the trees you smell are, in fact, essential oils they have breathed into the immediate atmosphere. During the road trip I shared with you through the Coconino National Forest in northern Arizona, the aroma of ponderosa pines was so strong that just opening the windows of our moving car caused us to relax, inhale deeply, and audibly sigh our contentment. If I had kept driving with simply a fleeting thought of "That smells nice," my family would still have received the benefits of deeper breaths and clearer, focused attention. However, stopping the car to acknowledge the amazing scent and share the exchange of life from one species to another with gratitude . . . well, now, that was a very different, sacred experience.

By our breathing in deeply through the nose, our parasympathetic ("rest and relaxation") nervous system is turned on. If you are stressed, just inhaling a long, deep breath through your nose can be very helpful. Doing this same exercise with an essential oil in the air (especially a scent you like!) will hasten the effects. Note that forest essential oils are not the only ones that have a beneficial response from the body.

Sometimes the respiratory system gets clogged or slowed down by allergies, illness, bacteria, or viruses, and, of course, bad air quality, such as pollutants and smoke. When the respiratory system slows down, the heart has to work harder and sometimes pump a little faster to get oxygen to the body. This task can be physically tiring if it is acute, and it is potentially dangerous if chronic. Several essential oils help support the respiratory system by loosening up mucus, reducing coughs, and reducing inflammation.

If thoughts are particularly busy or stuck on something, simply taking deep breaths is one of the easiest ways control the stress level held in the body. However, essential oils, through respiration, can also be beneficial. One of the simplest helpers that can be used for travel, in the car, packed in a bag, or left by the nightstand is a personal inhaler, also called

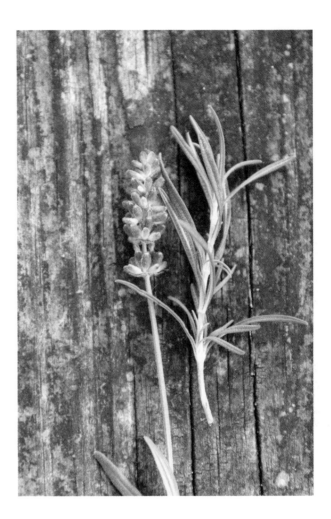

an aromastick or aromawand. Dropping a few oils into these little guys is convenient and easy (see "Ways to Use Essential Oils," pages 101–9). Using a personal necklace diffuser is another easy way to support breathing while being free from physical skin contact with an oil. Another hands-free option is to simply place a few drops on a cotton ball or tissue and place it near the intended user (not directly on wood or plastic, though). This is also a great way to provide access to essential oils to those who are bed bound, in an office where they are unable to run a diffuser, or traveling. Massage therapists have long used the trick of placing a single drop of eucalyptus

or lavender oil on a tissue and placing it near the face cradle to assist with relaxed, open breathing.

Diffusers are the top choice for assisting any respiratory issue. Breathing is much easier when you can allow the inhalation and exhalation to take place naturally. Due to their volatile nature, dispersing

If you are using a diffuser, please note that their most appropriate and safe use with essential oils is for a much shorter time than most diffusers run automatically. Best practices are 30 minutes on and 60 to 120 minutes off. Less time on is best for children, who benefit from as little as 10 to 20 minutes. Give your body a chance to readjust to the wonders of the essential oils. Plus, if you are constantly exposed to the same essential oils for many hours a day, day after day, there is a chance of developing a sensitivity to them (see page 97). Besides, your sense of smell can only detect the aromas for about 15 minutes before it goes into aromatic overload and shuts down. This becomes more of a concern for those who work in an industry, such as massage therapists, or for home users that love their diffuser so much they keep it running constantly. Rotate your oils, use intermittently, and give their internal and external alchemy a chance to make changes.

I suggest you start with three essential oils that your family enjoys—maybe lavender, sweet orange, and cypress or laurel. With these three oils, you can support the respiratory system in many ways, including mental calm and emotional lightness, and still have a variety of scents.

essential oils in a diffuser is one of the best means to support air quality, immunity support, and hence the well-being of the lungs. Not only will the air smell great, but the therapeutic benefits of the oils will affect any persons in the vicinity. David Crow mentioned ancient "community immunity" of aromatic plants has been modernized by essential oils with the use of diffusers.

# Smell

### THE OLFACTORY SYSTEM

How the brain uses essential oils is quite amazing. Bones were once thought of as being quite solid, but we now know they actually have a slight "give" and are porous, with openings that allow nutrients, blood, and oxygen to travel. Plus, there are openings in bones for tendons to secure the hinges of your moving parts. The skull, which protects your brain from harm, is not one solid cap but has tiny movements between its sutures, permitting adjustments to pressure, changes in altitude, and muscular movements. I like to think of it as bones having built-in breathing space.

The small bony plate that separates your nasal cavities and your brain is of particular interest here. Your nose is separated from your brain by a ¼-inch-thick piece of bone. It is filled with perforations to allow multiple exchanges from the outside world to have direct contact with your brain.

Unlike creatures that use other organs to detect fragrances, such as snakes that flick out their tongue to "taste" the odors of the air, humans use the internal features of the olfactory bulb, deep in the nose, just past the bony plate, nestled close to the brain. The sense of smell is the first sense to develop: babies are born with it in full swing (taste is also developed at birth), making it the oldest developed sense that the brain begins to process. But how do smells get past the bony plate?

Odors are chemical proteins, called odorants. In humans, these tiny chemicals enter the body via the inhalation of air. Your mouth actually helps you smell and your sense of smell helps you taste. Have you ever had a stuffy nose and not been able to taste your food? Conversely, tasting a scent in the air can indicate just how strong the particles are that

are floating around. However, your nose is the star player here.

Before anything even reaches the bony plate, odorants must travel past the fine hairs of the nostrils, which help prevent large particles, such as dust, from going into the airway, while small aromatic vapors can continue to travel. At the back of the nose is the magic gate to all the aromatic mystery, called the olfactory epithelium. There, the odorants are broken down by mucus that coats the inside of the nose. As they travel deeper into the nose, they begin to stimulate teeny-tiny nerve endings at the roof of the nose, called olfactory receptor cells. These hairlike nerve endings are like the string at the end of a balloon. These threads go upward into porous openings in the bony plate and are received by the olfactory bulb (this would be the balloon that the nerves are attached to).

The olfactory bulb begins to process the chemicals and sends signals to the brain based on the receptors' activation. An adult can pick up about 10,000 different scents, using 40,000,000 different receptor neurons (the only neurons in the body to renew themselves every 4 to 6 weeks). Different smells are triggered by different neurons in different combinations. The scent of bread, cheese, and tomato sauce will smell differently individually than all together as pizza. The receptors pick up the totality and bank the pieces of information based on the combination. A trained nose, however, may be able to distinguish subtle differences—such as whether this pizza had pepperoni or that pizza had a different

# INTEGRATIVE THERAPY

Humans are complex and often their health benefits from holistic support.

Sometimes that means the support has to be "out of the box," or as it is called in the medical field, alternative. Dr. R Adams Cowley founded the Shock Trauma Center in Baltimore, Maryland, years after he realized men in battle from the Korean War were dying not from their wounds but from the trauma and shock they were internalizing from their experience of *receiving* the wounds. He found that treating these mental and emotional symptoms saved more lives than conventional medical treatment alone. Now the University of Maryland successfully runs an Integrative Wellness Program overlapping supportive and alternative health care with Reiki, acupuncture, music therapy, art therapy, and, of course, aromatherapy. Scientific evidence documents the health shifts in each of these modalities. Such care is subjective; people's individual needs and overall well-being will determine which modality will resonate with them the most and how they will respond.

Donna Audia, team leader at the program, said that to help some of the younger patients (and adults) feel more relaxed in their hospital setting, they are given a choice of different essential oils (five to six to choose from) to sniff anytime they feel stressed or need to sleep. Options might include lime, orange, and lavender. Patients pick the one

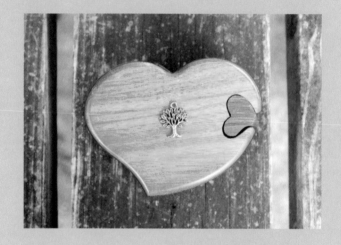

they like and are given a small, sealable container holding a cotton ball with a drop or two of the oil. The small gesture is often met with gratitude by parents. Donna emphasizes if people like what they smell, they are more apt to use the oil and experience its therapeutic benefits. Plus, inhaling through the nose helps induce the parasympathetic ("rest and rejuvenate") nervous system, which may also reduce anxiety.

The University of Arizona's Center for Integrative Medicine offers a college-level aromatherapy course designed by registered aromatherapist/herbalist Mindy Green, to educate medical staff, integrative practitioners, and the public in how essential oils can benefit the body, mind, emotions, and spirit.

kind of cheese. These chemicals are translated into pieces of information that then begin to travel along the olfactory tract. Kind of like catching the subway to the next destination, all the information from the scent goes along for the ride.

The neurons travel to different places within the brain, including the amygdala, thalamus, and neo-cortex. In other words, these chemicals have a direct line to the brain. Think about that for a second. Everything you smell goes straight to your brain. There is no filtering system where it changes form (whereas food goes through an entire digestive process to make it available to the bloodstream to get to the brain).

This immediate scent processing does not waste any time, kicking in the fight-or-flight response in times of danger, from the smell of smoke to the odor of a large predator too close for comfort. Smelling good food stimulates digestion even before a bite is tasted, and smell can even trigger a memory from the past (think of Proust's evocative scent of made-leines). Even Shakespeare mentions, "There's rose-mary, that's for remembrance." Science has since proven rosemary does indeed help with memory!

Because this nose-brain connection is so imme-diate, it is very important that you use true essential oils and not chemical synthetics designed to trick your sense of smell. The latter could potentially cause problems when your brain processes the mis-information thinking it is authentic natural aromas. Chemical fragrances of candles and cleaning materi-als, such as laundry soap, are not natural scents, but

the brain can be trained to like them—another rea-son to take care when selecting your essential oils.

Were there only one way to use essential oils, it could be through scent alone. Using personal inhal-ers and room diffusers can bring exponential ben-efits. A man in his forties who was going through stressful changes in his life agreed to participate in an experiment I offered, involving a custom blend of supportive essential oils. The blend needed to be something he would enjoy and therefore use. He mentioned he liked earthy smells as well as the ocean. Vetiver not only held the scent of earth I was looking for, but also the energetic principles suitable to the recipe—and I included laurel for a fresh top-mid note that would create the "open air" feeling of the seaside. And so "Earth and Sky" was born; you can find its recipe on page 274.

## Feeling

### THE LIMBIC SYSTEM
After the olfactory tract begins to deliver the infor-mation to the brain (think of the subway arriving at Grand Central Station), the limbic system takes over. It receives the new information and begins to match it to what it already has on file. This system asso-ciates smells and emotions with experiences, help-ing you retain memories of dangerous or pleasing events from the past. It also allows you to identify current information, such as immediately recogniz-ing the scent of a chocolate chip cookie anytime,

The sense of smell can be strengthened and "stretched" like a muscle. With careful attention, you can learn to smell layers of aromas within a single scent. For example, rose geranium has a wonderful roselike scent, but is also green, herbaceous, and slightly earthy.

Scent identification skills may depend on one's exposure. My husband's ability to discern certain papers and inks by smell was fine-tuned by his experience in the printing industry. Wine, tea, chocolate, and cheese connoisseurs as well as experienced chefs know the layers of fragrance of a good product will be an indicator of its taste. Essential oil scents have the same complexity, available to those who are interested in expanding their sense of smell.

Try this:

Pick your favorite essential oil. Look it up in Part 3 and read the description of its scent identifiers before you sniff. Open the bottle and place a drop on a tissue.

What do you smell first? That is the top note. Anything that you smell a few minutes to a few hours later is most likely going to change to a mid note. Base notes are slower to evaporate and will linger after the oil is dry. Smell it 24 hours later to distinguish the scent changes. Be patient if it all smells the same to you at first. You will find that your ability to recognize certain attributes grows with practice!

anywhere. This can work in your favor at times, and as a limitation at others.

The sense of smell associated with an experience can mean different things to different people. If my grandmother grew lavender in her garden and I loved going over to her house, loved Grandma, and always felt nurtured there, there's a pretty good chance I would always associate anything that smells like lavender with a positive experience (and with Grandma). However, if Grandma was a smoker (an odor association), neglected her house and me, I loathed visiting her, and the lavender in her yard drew bees, which frightened me, well, I'd likely instead associate the scent of lavender with unpleasant-smelling old ladies, neglect, mutual dislike, and maybe even fear. Because of the human processing within the limbic system, experiences can be very subjective, as can the introduction of the scent of essential oils.

The limbic system guides the internal forces of eating, sexual behavior, and sleep; in addition, emotions, instinctive drives, motivations, memories, and memory-triggered responses are all connected in some way to the relationship of scent and this system. Several parts of the brain make up the total function of the limbic system, much like a community coming together to get a big job done, where each part has an important individual role, but you only really see the full effects once all the parts are in motion.

The *amygdala* is a bit of an emotional gatekeeper, processing incoming information and

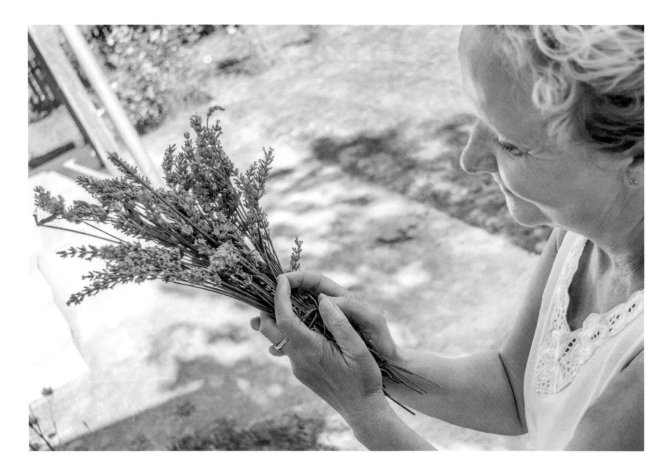

deciding whether it is a threatening/stressful force or a pleasurable one. Any potential danger signals trigger the *hypothalamus* to respond with hormones or physical shifts (e.g., running away). If there are enough triggers of emotional pain, fear, or distress—e.g., if certain scents are associated with stress and exposure is frequent or prolonged—the brain begins to make physical changes in its actual structure, called lesions. Lesions can affect future emotional processing, creating a self-protectively dulled or nonemotional connection to an experience. Worse yet, the information can make its way to the permanent files of memory. This can be hard to overcome once it is "hardwired," so to speak.

This is just as important when an experience is amazing. For instance, I recall the scent of plume-

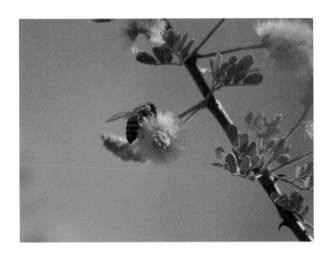

internal functions of the endocrine system (hormones), the autonomic system (regulatory systems, such as digestion, heartbeat, and breath), and the emotional context of the limbic system all begin to express in the physical body, mind, and spirit with illness and chemical imbalances. This is important to consider in women's health, especially with regard to hormones and experiences that are in flux throughout childbearing years.

The *septum*'s job is to maintain peace; that is to say, to regulate aggressive tendencies if the amygdala tries to go into a panic. The limbic system has built-in checks and balances, but they can be overridden and conditioned. That is why being told something over and over again can be uplifting, as in the case of affirmations, or devastating, as with verbal abuse. The brain literally begins to associate the conditioning with the experience. Basically, the brain is constantly learning from your behaviors and experiences and responds accordingly. The response then becomes conditioned. I'm sure you've noticed people who always seem to look at the bright side of life, even on a cloudy day, whereas others act as if every day is a thunderstorm.

Essential oils are a very important noninvasive helper in breaking habits of negative conditioning. The olfactory receptors receive the information of bright, beautiful sunshine metabolized in the life of a sweet orange by way of its essential oil, whose chemistry has an uplifting, anxiety-reducing, and antidepressant effect on the limbic system. The appropriate choice of essential

rias with fondness because their allure was what I first smelled getting off a plane and upon entering the airport in Maui, Hawaii. The thrill of where I was became linked inextricably with the fragrance of that particular plant; had I smelled a different plant as I stepped off that plane, it would probably be the one I associate with Maui instead.

A series of events in the brain creates movement of our hormones, internal temperatures, body fluid balances, and even appetite control and steroid release. Insomnia can be connected to the part of the limbic system that the hypothalamus is in charge of in determining the input of circadian rhythm support. The hypothalamus's whole job is to maintain a state of internal harmony called homeostasis. Homeostasis is important in maintaining balance, whether the body and mind are under stress or doing fine. If the incoming information throws off the homeostasis on a continual basis, the

> Try this:
> Think of an experience in your past that had a favorable scent to it. For instance, I fondly associate my great-grandmother's house with the aromas of food served when the entire family gathered. What emotions relate to your choice of recollection?
>
> Now create a new memory. Gather two or three essential oils in front of you. After holding each bottle, closed, mindfully choose one to open—only one. Gently waft the scent under your nose, allow your lips to soften into a relaxed smile, and think to yourself, "This is a beautiful moment."
>
> Tomorrow, do the same. And the next day. Do this once a day, every day, for a week (or two). Then, give it a break. After a week or two, open the bottle and see whether your mind and heart automatically go to the thought and emotion of "This is a beautiful moment."

oils can be very supportive of the septum's job of maintaining peace.

Remember my drive through the pine forest in Arizona? The scent of pine, associated with the memory of lightness and openness, is a good choice to have in my home resources; as a matter of fact, I even diffused a little pine the other day while writing this book, to lighten up the atmosphere in the office. It worked! My limbic system immediately responded favorably with deep breaths and memories of that long, open stretch of highway, while the aroma of pine was soothing to my nervous system. My family members benefited from the antimicrobial actions in the clean air.

Other factors change the limbic system's processing of scent, emotion, and memory: age, where you live (near the ocean or atop of a mountain), the culture you were brought up with and the one you currently reside with, as well as past associations with scents. During pregnancy and breastfeeding, women may find their sense of smell increases (sometimes overwhelmingly so) as an innate, instinctual protective awareness of the environment, and perhaps to be keenly in tune with the scents of the baby. This is called hyperosmia.

Sometimes, the connection of scent and emotion are not as clear, as in the case of anosmia (loss of the sense of smell), which can result from head injury, a virus, atrophy to the olfactory bulb, or a possible congenital issue. With minor temporary disruptions of smell, as with the common cold, smelling essential oils can assist in reducing inflammation of sinuses and loosening up mucus. The big question with scent loss, temporary or permanent, is whether oils work if you cannot smell them. The answer is yes. The chemical constituents can still do their job; although, the limbic system does not connect the pleasurable sensations associated with the scent. However, using essential oils may help some people retrain the olfactory bulb to fire neurons to make the connection if physical processes to do so are still available. It's not an exact science and no claims can be made that it absolutely works. "Smell is unpredictable," when approached this way, cautions David Crow, "but occasionally, a scent makes it through enough to be identified" (2016).

## The Skin

### THE INTEGUMENTARY SYSTEM

The protective layer of the skin is the first line of defense in keeping the body healthy. Bacteria, fungi, viruses, excess water and other fluids, heat and cold, and wind are all shielded from penetrating the inner body with the many layers of this flexible organ, the largest in the body. Skin also keeps hydration inside the body and prevents necessary system changes from being exposed to the atmosphere.

Skin can change color as a signal and sign of change and distress; for instance, sunburns and rashes can signal external and internal changes, indicating attention is needed. Actual irritation or abrasion of the skin can show up immediately. Ingesting a substance that the body reacts to as allergenic may also change the appearance and sensations of the skin (think: hives). If skin is too dry or too oily, this may signal that something within the system is out of balance. Observing the skin can help in choosing an essential oil.

Essential oils cannot eradicate nutritional deficiencies or allergies; however, they can provide beautiful support for regenerative and anti-inflammatory conditions, such as wound healing.

The skin can also give feedback on the emo-

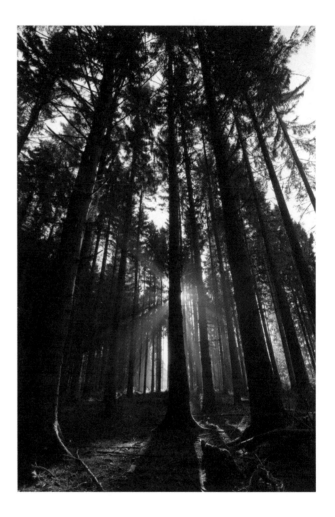

tional and mental states connected to the limbic system. A person's face may flush due to the emotion of embarrassment, but someone else may turn red due to overexertion or anger. Conversely, one may go pale due to shock, when the internal organs have kicked in to handle immediate pro-

# STORY THYME

This complex memory-scent-emotion association is why experiences with certain scents are so personal. When I decided to develop my scent observation skills, I gained a fondness for many essential oils that I'd initially rejected. Before, if the scent did not fall into an easy-to-identify category of "familiar and likable," it was laid by the wayside.

But something mysterious happens if you allow yourself to be curious, not judgmental. For example, it may be helpful to place an aroma in a greater context, such as knowing which part or stage of life of the plant is represented in the scent.

Take the smell of earth. Desert storms are magical; they literally open up the arid floor, hydrating the crevices, and the earth releases a breath of coming alive, an awakening. I experienced these storms while growing up in southern Arizona. As a child, I just interpreted their odor as wet dirt. As an adult, I understand that precious microbes held within the soil are activated once hydrated and nutrients for fertile support of plants become available. The scent of the earth also combines with the fragrance of all the other plants quenched by a deep soak all the way down to their subterranean roots.

My appreciation for this after-the-rain scent of earth has certainly changed my impression of the

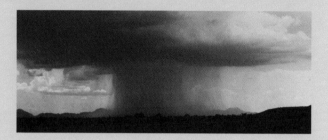

smell of dirt, which I now call terrain, soil, or earth, depending on the scent exchange. It most certainly has opened me to be curious about vetiver, which comes from the roots of *Vetiveria zizanoides* grass, not from dirt, but of it, and which many say smells like dirt. Once I'd tapped into the "real" aroma of the soil, vetiver did not smell like dirt at all. Instead, it is slightly woody and warm, and has an underlying sweetness hidden in the fragrance, and a whisper of greenness. As you might expect, its use can be grounding.

Here is one more thought to further expand your visual-emotive-scent connection to earthy aromas. In India, the first rain to break the drought season is revered by gathering the mud from the first downpour and distilling it, along with sandalwood, to create a very special cocreation thought to capture the scent of rain, which is the connection of earth (receiving) and sky (releasing).

cessing of blood flow for survival. These are not primary functions of the skin, but expressions of it in connection with other systems. These expressions are valid in observing the alchemy of an experience.

Having a bit of knowledge on how the skin works, what it does, and how to aid it, will be beneficial in picking essential oils and the most appropriate method of application.

Basic functions of the skin as a functioning organ include:

- *Protection:* The skin protects both internally and externally (keeps things out, such as rain; and keeps things in, such as the body's hydration).
- *Permeability:* The skin both inhibits and allows fluid, oxygen, and carbon dioxide exchange in appropriate provisions. (Absorption is allowed through the many layers of the skin, but prevented from instant access to internal organs.)
- *Temperature regulation:* Maintaining proper temperature is important to the health of the human body. Fevers and heat-induced activities are cooled by sweat and evaporation through the skin. Cold temperatures are prevented from cooling the internal organs by the skin's defending them against exposure.
- *Waste regulation:* The skin removes toxins from the body via sweat.
- *Sensory input:* Skin is the largest organ to send messages to the brain via the central nervous system when stimulated by touch, pressure,

### TEARS

Tears protect the eyes and amend and connect with physical, mental, and emotional conditions. The body produces three different kinds of tears: reflex, continuous, and emotional. According to Judith Orloff, MD, tears vary in the amount of hormones, enzymes, and water they contain. Reflex tears, which can be triggered by smelling something with strong vapors, flush out the eyes. This may occur if essential oils are placed too close to the eyes or nose—another reason to handle essential oils safely! Continuous tears lubricate the eye; emotional tears release stress hormones that help regulate the body.

heat, and cold, which can be perceived as pain or pleasure.

- *Feedback:* Internal alchemic changes due to emotions, mental stresses, and nutritional requirements and lack thereof are expressed in the skin conditions.

Listening to a wordless organ is quite a task. The holistic approach taught in most alternative care methods, such as massage therapy, acupuncture, and chiropractic, as well as the professional skin services of an esthetician or energetic training of a Reiki master, all include being aware of the skin's communication of the body's ability to regulate the processes of the outside world and the internal alchemy. As a massage therapist, I appreciate Madame Maury's approach (see page 29) to observe and recognize each individual's expressions and combination of experiences that the person brings to a session.

## Skin Layers

The skin consists of many individual layers, most often grouped as three major layers: the epidermis, the dermis, and the subcutaneous layer.

*The epidermis:* This is the top layer, the one you see and make physical contact with. *Epi* means "before, on, over, or after"; and *dermis,* "skin." There are five layers to the epidermis, including the layer of dead skin cells that, having completed the entire process of the epidermis's purpose, have been pushed up to the edge of the skin universe to be released. The body naturally sloughs off these cells, but brushing up against the skin, or exfoliation, also eliminates these cells (see sidebar). The next four layers (which have layers within themselves!) gradually move from the bottom to the top of the epidermis to effect cellular rejuvenation. A full skin cell cycle from cell birth to completion takes 5 to 6 weeks, which is why skin care products suggest using for 6 to 8 weeks to see results.

*The dermis:* The largest, fully functional, all-living cellular tissue of the skin is the dermis layer. It is responsible for skin's color, its elasticity through

The oldest layers of the skin are what you can flake off easily simply by scratching with a fingernail. These skin cells are no longer living. Most people are familiar with the practice of exfoliation, which removes dead skin cells from the surface to expose the newer skin layers, stimulating cellular rejuvenation and reducing the appearance of unhealthy, dull, or clogged pores. Fresh skin is more open to penetration by topical products. However, constantly skimming off the top layer reduces the buffer to the layers of skin containing naturally protective secretions and bacteria-fighting enzymes. In other words, it is important to have clean, refreshed skin, but overcleaning it can stimulate the body's need to protect it. This can lead to excess oil production to lubricate it, or to excessive dryness if the natural oils are unable to replenish properly. Supporting the skin based on its needs and ability to create harmony on its own is important. For example, acne is sometimes better approached by cleansing with facial oils or creams that contain antimicrobial and cellular-rejuvenating essential oils, in proper dilution, rather than with soaps or detergents that strip the skin (often causing more oil production, exacerbating the situation).

connective tissue, as well as hydration, blood, and lymphatic circulation; oil production through sebaceous glands; sweat excretion; and sheltering the nerve endings that communicate much of our sense of touch. Whew! A lot happens here.

The hair follicle in the dermis layer of the skin is connected to the only muscle within the skin. The arrector pili muscle is responsible for the movement of hairs standing on end and lying flat against the skin. Movements of the arrector pili are excited by temperature changes of cold and emotions, such as fear. Those who believe in energetic sensitivities also attribute reactions to unseen electrical currents undetected by other obvious means.

The dermis also contains the hair follicles, each of which holds an individual hair that moves up from the protected inner dermis layer to the outside world. It is believed that between dermal cells and through the hair follicles, external substances enter the skin to travel to the nerve, blood, and lymphatic layers of the body. It is important to note that follicle-free areas, such our palms and the soles of our feet, indicate there is a lessened likelihood of penetration of external substances into the bloodstream in these areas. These areas still have access to an incredible network of highly available capillaries through the skin, so massaging the entire hand and foot has physical benefits of increasing circulation on reflex points, but also through absorption in the more porous locations nearby.

The dermal layer can be reached with proper dilution of essential oils and other products, but it is important to follow specific safety instructions with open wounds, cuts, and burns. Learn to recog-

nize when a wound needs medical attention, such as stitches. A lot of bodily systems are exposed once the dermal layer is involved. Infection is not a welcome guest. Get to know your antibacterial, antimicrobial, antiviral, and skin-rejuvenating essential oils, such as lavender, Roman and German chamomiles, helichrysum, frankincense, sandalwood, and cedarwood.

*The subcutaneous layer:* Meaning "below the skin," in plants this layer is called the hypodermis, which has the same definition. In humans, it is a protective layer of cushioning of fat that acts a shock absorber to protect organs and bones, and also provides the body with insulation, helping maintain the appropriate temperature within all the bodily systems. Within this layer, arteries and capillaries bring the blood supply to the dermis. Essential oils that help protect and support broken capillaries, such as helichrysum, need to reach this layer.

## The Muscular and Nervous Systems

I am placing these two systems together, although they are equally important individually, as the former is directly dependent upon the signals sent by the latter. The muscular system allows for movement of the physical body, providing flexibility, strength, and stamina. The nervous system sends and receives signals from all systems in the body to the central nervous system to the brain, but also has

Massage therapists are trained to do very light massage to stimulate the gentle flow of the lymphatic system. If pressure goes too deeply, stimulation of blood flow into the muscles is activated. If you decided to use massage to stimulate your lymphatic system, remember that the pressure only has to go as deep as the second major layer of skin to make a difference. That's pretty light. Think of the weight of a nickel balancing on your fingertip. Those who believe that deep tissue pressure is the only way to go are missing out on some pretty profound results in the softest, gentlest of massages. If you decide to try this, remember to stroke toward the heart and the center of the torso.

an emotional component with a direct connection to pain perception and muscular contraction.

The human muscular system has more than 600 muscles, 14 major muscle groups, and about 4,000 tendons, but that number varies according to which muscle group is involved. Muscles are unique in the human body in having the ability to change form (get bigger or smaller) depending on the amount they are used. They retract to their original shape after being stretched, contracted, rotated, depleted, or overused. The elasticity of muscles and the movement of the body is dependent on the overall health of the body, proper nutrition, and sleep, but the muscles' responses to stimuli outside the body

(touch) and inside the body (brain) are solely due to the nervous system.

The nervous system, intricate and complex, has 12 pairs of nerves attached to the brain (each pair includes the left and the right side of the brain and body) and 31 pairs attached to the spinal cord, branching off into smaller and smaller plexus stages as they go from larger areas (shoulders, arms) to smaller areas (hands, fingers). The intricacy of the final points of the nerves that meet at the dermis layer of the skin send signals of pressure, touch, temperature, and distress or disruption.

When the nervous system is stressed, the muscular system begins to respond by contracting, bracing the immediate area in an effort to protect that part of the body, like a shield. Conversely, if nerves have been damaged and cannot send a signal indicating the stress, the muscle cannot defend the area, leaving it limp and unresponsive.

Essential oils can soothe both muscles and nerves. A blend of Roman chamomile, lavender, and peppermint accomplish both at the same time.

Ginger and black pepper can help bring in warmth to cold areas of nerve and muscle sensations, whereas eucalyptus can be cooling. Nervine (nerve-soothing) essential oils are especially helpful for bruised trauma or muscle fatigue. Helichrysum, known as one of the top skin healers, also has properties of nervine action. Nervines can also relieve nervous anxiety or feeling overwhelmed. Laurel and cypress, due to their grounded, contractive quality, bring energy into a person rather than its being

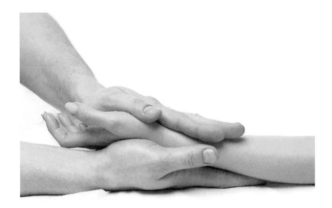

scattered, especially when diffused or used in a personal inhaler. Used in a warm massage oil, cypress also adds astringent qualities known in Oriental medicine as purifying the blood, according to acupuncturist and aromatherapist Gabriel Mojay, and its ability to help regulate blood acts as an antispasmodic for muscular pain (1997). Laurel also acts as an antispasmodic essential oil upon the muscles, but is best for cramping issues and cold stagnation.

## Other Systems

The endocrine and digestive systems are two additional significant and principal players in human well-being.

### THE ENDOCRINE SYSTEM

This system includes the hypothalamus, pituitary, pineal, thyroid, and thymus glands as well as the pancreas, each secreting its respective hormones into the body that affect sleep, sexual functions, reproduction and the function of reproductive organs, metabolism, how fast we grow and develop, and our mood. The delicate balance of these hormones have some hand in every other bodily system's response. For instance, hormones secreted in excess or in extreme deficiency can produce symptoms ranging from PMS to diabetes.

Clearly maintaining proper hormone function and correcting hormonal imbalances are beyond the capacity of essential oils. If you have symptoms that lead you to believe that you have a hormone problem, you should consult your primary care physician and/or an endocrinologist. You also may benefit from consulting a qualified professional in the field of endobiogeny, a systematic approach to finding balance among nerves, hormones, and organ systems that sometimes includes aromatherapy.

Essential oils can assist in soothing and calming some of the effects of an out-of-balance endocrine system until the internal issues are medically or nutritionally resolved properly. For instance, cramping due to PMS can be relieved with gentle abdominal massage with a little lavender, clary sage, or perhaps some geranium in the mixture. Nervous anxiety or mood fluctuations accompanying hormonal swings or sleep disruptions can be assisted by breathing in the scents of lavender, sweet orange, clary sage, or rose. Deep earthy scents of patchouli, vetiver, or frankincense can be helpful for those feeling a bit scattered or ungrounded.

To reiterate, while diagnosis of a disorder or major system concern is not something within the scope of the home user, essential oils' stress-relief properties are certainly helpful when trying to get a major body system under control and harmonized.

## THE DIGESTIVE SYSTEM

The digestive system, or gut, is considered an "open" system because, at its start and finish, there is an opening to the outside world. Scientifically speaking, there are two parts to the gastrointestinal (GI) tract: hollow organs and solid ones. The open organs are the esophagus, stomach, both the small and large intestines, colon, rectum, and anus, all of which foods pass through during consumption and digestion. The solid organs are the liver, pancreas, and gallbladder, which help further the process and metabolize the nutrients, getting them ready for absorption from the intestines. Everything you eat is either stored, expelled, or used as energy. This includes energy for your brain. If you feed your body junk, you feed your brain junk.

The most recent discovery is what is being referred to as "the second brain." The enteric nervous system within the digestive system works independently of the central nervous system of the brain and spinal cord. However, the systems are connected by the vagus nerve, the longest cranial nerve that connects to the gut. The vagus nerve communicates to the brain information based on

Clinical aromatherapists have extensive training in using aromatherapy for specific medical concerns and take consideration of every facet of the circumstances with a person's needs: physical or mental concerns, contraindications, any possible medicine interactions, purpose of use, duration of use, method of application, how open is the person to using aromatherapy, and other supportive methods to recommend. They do not diagnose, but can support complicated concerns with a mindful and educated approach. Be mindful: Some people call themselves essential oil "coaches" or "wellness representatives." This does not mean they have had any formal training, nor does it mean they are trained in aromatherapy. Qualified clinical or certified aromatherapists study essential oils, connect to the safe use of stress reduction, and follow best practices.

the different flora present in the gut. The brain then responds to this information. While this kind of relay action works well in the central nervous system by signaling to retreat in response to pain, the enteric nervous system and the brain do not communicate in this same way. UCLA researchers confirmed in 2013 that mood and stress are affected by the signals sent from the gut to the brain, not the other way around (Foster 2013). Methods of well-being used in Ayurveda have long established the gut is key to the health of the mind and the emotional heart.

Why is this important for essential oil users to know? Phytonutrients are vital for stress relief of the physical body and for the brain's processing of healthy emotions. Smelling essential oils can help with emotions and can ease discomfort with gentle abdominal massage, but if digestion itself is poorly attended to, the oils will produce, at best, only temporary relief.

On the plus side, for thousands of years aromatic plants have triggered the digestion system to begin the process of getting ready for food before it enters the body, simply through scent. This information can be very useful in several ways:

*Appetite stimulation:* Warm, spicy scents of culinary herbs—try fennel or cardamom—in a diffuser, personal inhaler, or just smelling from the bottle do nicely.

*Nausea:* Try ginger or peppermint in a personal inhaler.

*Bloating or gas:* Massage the abdomen in a clockwise motion with a drop of two of fennel, peppermint, or ginger in a carrier oil. (Do not use if pregnant. For children, use lavender or Roman chamomile instead).

## Spiritual

Spiritual experiences have been marked with ritual and ceremony—raw and primal or tightly controlled—using aromatic plants for eons. Certain scents and aromatic plants, such as frankincense, have been recorded as being associated with ritual and ceremony well into antiquity. However, spirituality is as subjective and personal as essential oils. That is, while we can agree mostly on the properties of an essential oil, ultimately the experience will be unique to the user. The same goes for spiritual endeavors.

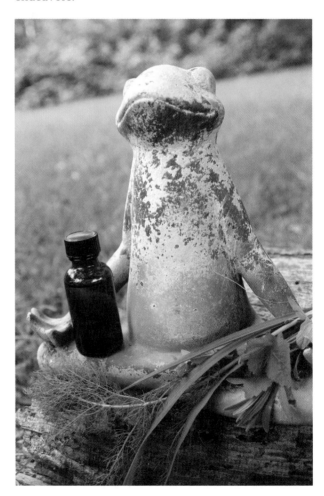

After distillation of essential oils became available, an aromatic plant that was once only available in season—or as twigs or branches burned in smudge sticks or bonfires or resins harvested from trees—could be enjoyed in the comfort of one's home. Although any scent could be used in meditative or other ceremonial practices, depending on your scent-emotive-memory connection, some historically recorded essential oils may deepen your experience of the spiritual space.

Using essential oils to break up stagnant energy and/or heavy feelings in a room, or to prepare a room for something special, is easy and encouraged. Diffusing lavender 30 minutes before going to bed, then turning off the diffuser before snuggling under the covers, is a lovely way to create a sacred and relaxing ritual for sleep.

Done in conjunction with reading, yoga, meditation, prayer, quiet movements of tai chi, or simply coloring an image to relax, smelling essential oils straight from the bottle, in a personal inhaler, or diffusing them for 30 minutes can be a wonderful treat for your well-being.

*For quiet meditation:* frankincense, sandalwood, lavender, cistus, or palo santo

*For a clear head and to "open up" the environment:* sweet orange, lavender, lemongrass, grapefruit, or laurel

*For reflective spaces to cope with an emotional day:* bergamot, mandarin, vetiver, lavender or clary sage, and cypress

*To quiet the mind at the end of the day:* sandal-

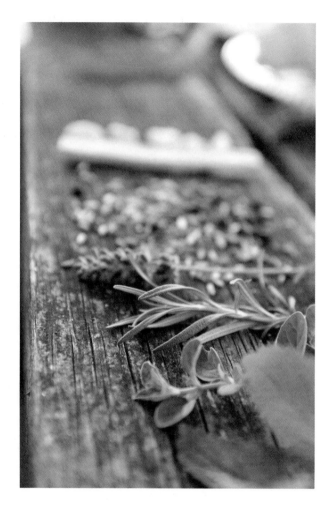

wood, lemongrass, sweet orange, vetiver, patchouli, lavender, marjoram, frankincense, or palo santo

*To alleviate fears and calm anxiety:* Roman chamomile, lavender, rose geranium, ginger, laurel, patchouli, pine, mandarin, sweet orange, vetiver, and ylang-ylang

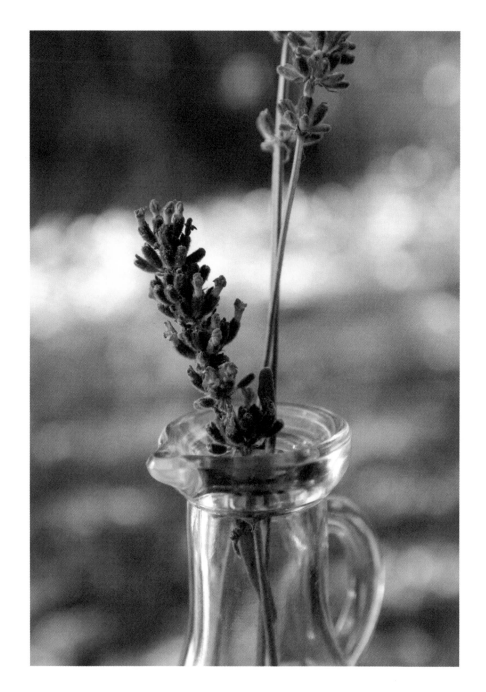

*For grounding:* vetiver, ginger (both are roots)

*For a broken heart:* rose, clary sage, lavender, frankincense, sandalwood, palo santo, helichrysum, laurel, or jasmine

*For depression:* sweet orange, patchouli, grapefruit, lemongrass, geranium, rose, ginger, frankincense, sandalwood, mandarin, or pine

## How Essential Oils Are Processed in the Body

Essential oil researcher Robert Tisserand has written an easy-to-follow account of the metabolization of essential oils. Simply put, inhalation of its aroma is the fastest way to benefit from an essential oil (2016).

Why? Inhalation of essential oils split the chemical information into two places: the brain and the lungs. According to Tisserand, approximately 5% goes to the brain and 95% enters the lungs via inhalation. Both the brain and lungs have access to the bloodstream. The bloodstream, liver, kidneys, and bladder all play a part in moving an inhaled vapor's chemicals through the body; the chemicals are then eliminated.

On the other hand, per Tisserand, when an oil is mixed with a lotion, gel, or carrier oil that gets massaged into the skin, some of the vapors will be inhaled as described. However, only about 5% of the

**MYTH: ESSENTIAL OILS CONTAIN HORMONES, VITAMINS, MINERALS, AND HELP OXYGENATE THE BODY.**

There are neither human hormones, nor vitamins, nor minerals in essential oils. Oils do have plant-based chemical components, but none falls into any of those categories. Nor does the body obtain oxygen from essential oils. While they do include oxygen within their molecular makeup, that does not in any way translate to oxygenating the human body. Humans do bring in more oxygen by taking deep breaths while smelling essential oils!

essential oils actually reach the muscles to find their way to the bloodstream. As during inhalation, once the oil's chemicals are in the bloodstream, the liver processes and metabolizes them and they move on to the kidneys and bladder to be eliminated.

Why is the liver involved? Because essential oils are nonnutritive—that is to say, they contain no nutritional value to the body—they must be processed out. Tisserand explains that the oils "are treated as xenobiotics, [meaning] foreign substances, and are detoxified by enzymes in the liver so they can be efficiently excreted."

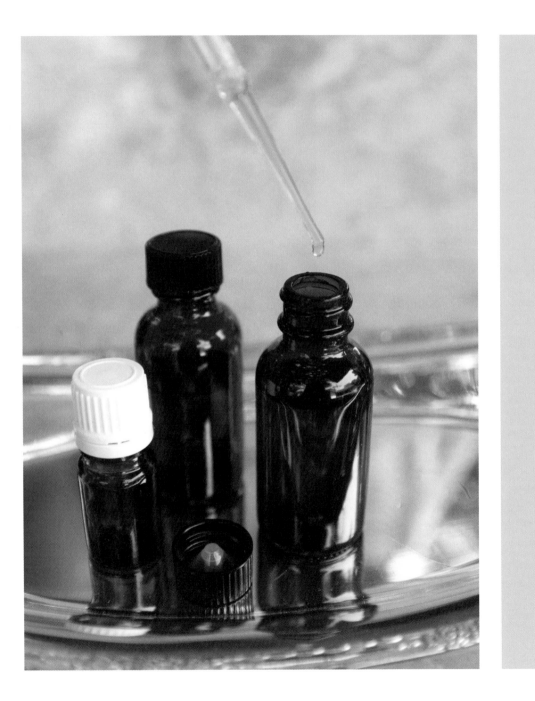

# Safety

**2**

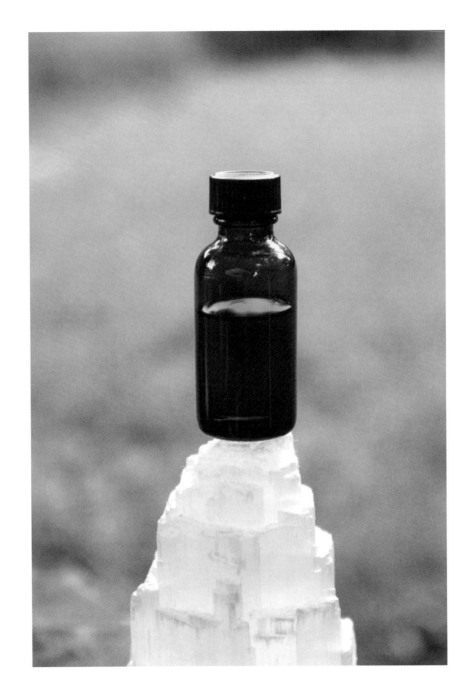

# CHAPTER 5

# Safety Guides, Reminders, and Precautions

*Adopt the pace of nature: her secret is patience.*
—Ralph Waldo Emerson

This is one of the most important chapters in the book.

Essential oils are 50 to 100 times more concentrated than in the plant, according to Robert Tisserand, co-author of *Essential Oil Safety*; therefore safety precautions apply differently than if you were using the plant source in its entirety or even as an herbal extract, tincture, or tea. Please use essential oils with patience, holding back the urge to add too many drops, and be aware of the individual needs of the recipient.

## Housekeeping Rules Concerning Essential Oils

These are precious oils requiring care. They are not so delicate that they go rancid, as may your cooking oils. As a matter of fact, pure essential oils do *not* go rancid; they are by nature antibacterial. However, some oils may oxidize; also, any water-based products they are placed in will begin to support bacteria in a short amount of time, if not processed to preserve, and even they should be used in a reasonable time frame. These include lotions, creams, gels, and hydrosols.

The following notes will help keep your essential oils happier and your body happier about using them.

### SHELF LIFE

Essential oils do have a shelf life, some longer than others. Those wonderful top-note citrus essential oils have some of the shortest usable life spans, whereas those deep base notes of patchouli seem to get bet-

# SAFETY GUIDE

Essential oils are both powerful and subtle. If you are unsure about appropriate use of an essential oil or blend on yourself or someone else or in a particular setting, consult a qualified aromatherapist. Aromatherapists have the necessary knowledge, experience, and training specifically for the the chemicals and contraindications of essential oils. Unless your doctor has had training specifically in aromatherapy, they might not be aware of certain reasons or safety concerns with essential oils. Use a doctor for medical diagnosis. Use an aromatherapist for essential oil safety information. Create a relationship with both your doctor and aromatherapist to best support your health.

Please practice safely, mindfully, and with the dual intentions to relieve stress and do no harm. Even if you are sure that you are using appropriate essential oils in the right way, be aware of rashes or other subtler reactions. Do not guess when it comes to essential oil safety.

Here are some key safety rules:

- Always dilute essential oils in a carrier oil.
- Babies, children, pregnant or nursing women, the elderly, very sick people, and pets are especially vulnerable to adverse effects from the incorrect or inappropriate use of essential oils.

Be sure to seek advice from a qualified aromatherapist as well as your medical doctor.

- Store essential and carrier oils away from heat and light, and in proper containers at proper temperatures. Amber (brown) or cobalt (blue) glass bottles are light safe and recommended for essential and carrier oils. The less air in the bottle's headspace (the area between the product and the cap), the better.
- Keep all essential oils away from the eyes and mucous membranes.
- Do not take essential oils internally.
- Avoid synthetic fragrances or oils. Use only authentic essential oils.
- More does not equal better! Refer to Chapter 15 for the correct dosages of drops. Refer to Part 3 for individual oil cautions and important notes.
- Use proper ventilation for the area in which essential oils will be used.
- Keep bottles away from pets and children. Curious little fingers, mouths, and paws need to be out of reach of all essential oils.
- Diffuse intermittently: 30 minutes on, 60 to 120 minutes off (for young children 10 to 15 minutes is plenty).
- Rotate oil use to prevent sensitization.

ter with age! The following are helpful ways to know which oil has which shelf life:

- Mark your bottle with the date of purchase. You may not be able to track when the batch of the oil was distilled, but you can keep track of how long you have had it on your personal shelf (many only have a shelf life of 12 months; others, a couple of years).
- If you can track its bottle's exact batch number to the distributor, you can learn how old the oil is. Be mindful that sale-priced oils may be an indication the retailer needs them to be purchased soon to ensure a reasonable shelf life. Purchase these only if you know you will be using them within a short period of time. (Order sample-size oils if you want to try one out inexpensively, instead of oils on sale.)
- The life span of some essential oils, such as citrus, conifers, or lavender, can be extended a bit longer or slowed by adding a drop of vitamin E. Vitamin E is an antioxidant (not a preservative).
- If you are familiar with the chemical makeup of each essential oil, you can get an idea of its shelf life expectancy, given proper storage, but that takes a bit more study and education.

## PROPER STORAGE

- A refrigerator is the ideal storage location; if that is not feasible, keep your oils in a cool, dark cabinet. (Citruses, conifers, and lavender are best in the fridge.)
- Always store away from direct sunlight and heat sources, as both can shorten oils' life span.

### MYTH: USING ESSENTIAL OILS EQUALS AROMATHERAPY.

Essential oils can be used for a multitude of purposes, including in cleaning supplies, toothpaste, lotions, and cosmetics. Adding oils merely for flavor or fragrance generally does not constitute aromatherapy.

Aromatherapy uses particular essential oils or blends specifically to benefit the body, mind, emotions, or spirit. The intentional use of these concentrated volatile oils can have subtle and profound effects on the body in ways that are neither tracked by the conscious mind nor immediately recognized by the emotions. Deeper still, spiritual aspects tend to be unique experiences for each individual. How will you know how an essential oil will affect you? You won't. The experience is very personal. Additionally, essential oils are scientifically documented to create a particular response and yet are subjectively variable depending on the person and his or her needs. Essential oils are, in essence, an exact inexact science and art—there is no "one size fits all" in aromatherapy.

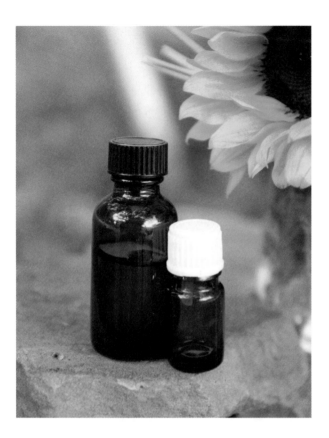

high-density polyethylene (HDPE) plastic (marked with a "2" for recycling in the US) will work as well.

- Keep essential oils in the smallest container they will fit into. If you ordered a ½-ounce (15 ml) bottle, but only half is left in the bottle (you'll most likely only need 5 ml), it would be better to transfer the remaining oil to a smaller bottle, to reduce the amount of headspace, so there won't be as much air/oxygen at the top of the bottle. Remember, air, heat, and light degrade an oil's integrity faster.
- Try not to use droppers, which hold air in the bottle, plus they pump air in and out of the essential oil every time you use them. Use droppers in small bottles if the mixture has been blended with a carrier and will be used in a reasonable amount of time, otherwise the oxygen may speed up the oxidation process.
- Keep away from children and pets. Children might drink essential oils or have adverse reactions to spills on their skin. Read the precautions concerning each kind of oil and note that these are powerful botanical chemical components; they do have a potential for harm if applied in too high a dilution or used improperly with children. Pets do not metabolize the essential oils the same way as humans (see sidebar "Your Pets Are Not Human," page 95).

- Store in amber (brown) or cobalt (blue) glass bottles.
- Never store essential oils in plastic containers—oils will degrade the plastic, contaminating the oil, and the container will lose its integrity.
- PET containers are the only acceptable hard plastic container to hold a blend that includes a carrier (see Chapter 15). Some report that

# YOUR PETS ARE NOT HUMAN

Dogs and cats do not metabolize essential oils the same way as humans. In some cases, oils can create more harm than good. Before I understood its effect on animals, I began to notice a pattern every time I diffused any oil from the *Melaleuca* genus, such as tea tree or niaouli: my dog would get lethargic and my cat would vomit. They were both reacting to the oil in the air. Precautions are mandatory with our furry, feathered, and scaled friends that cannot communicate verbally.

For safety's sake, do not use any essential oils, especially via diffusers, around pets in confined areas, terrariums, fish tanks, or ponds. Cats especially lack an enzyme in their liver that prevents metabolization of essential oils. Remember, in the natural world, small amounts of essential oils are released to deter or attract specific species interaction. Pets cannot escape the natural deterrent if in a closed house or room or body of water. If you must use indoors, provide proper ventilation—pets must have access to fresh air—or remove the animals from the room completely. Separate pets into another room if you are diffusing and air it out before allowing them to come back into the room. Investigate the specifics concerning your pets from a properly trained animal aromatherapist (yes, there are some out there!) or your veterinarian. Note: Not all vets have been properly trained for safe application of essential oils on pets.

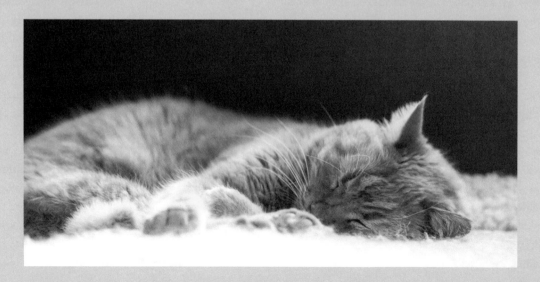

| In case of an emergency: stay calm. | | |
| --- | --- | --- |
| **INGESTION** | **SKIN** | **EYES** |
| 1. If ingested, especially by children, dilute immediately by drinking milk (2% or full-fat milk is best). Do not drink water. Do not induce vomiting. 2. Call poison control. | 1. Dilute immediately by applying a carrier oil (not water) to the skin. 2. Wash with copious amounts of soap and rinse with water. | 1. Wipe gently with vegetable carrier oil (coconut oil, jojoba, etc.) on a cotton ball or soft washcloth. Do not rinse with water (water spreads the oil). 2. Repeat as necessary. 3. Thoroughly wash with water as a final rinse. |

## Oxidation

Chemicals that are volatile (that turn quickly from a liquid to a vapor) produce the aromas you smell first; they also tend to have a shorter shelf life. They remind me of effervescence: bubbles that rise quickly to the top, and if exposed to the air for too long, go flat. In the case of essential oils, the "flat" part is usually oxidation and a loss of therapeutic integrity and aroma. Oxidation is when exposure to air alone creates a change in the chemistry of an oil. You may know it as the process that makes your apples and avocados turn brown once they are cut open. Some essential oils show oxidation by getting sticky around the cap or changing scent or color. This is not the case for all oils, so it is important to know the shelf life of each oil and store them properly. Oxidized oils lose therapeutic value and can cause skin irritation and adverse reactions. Therefore, do not use oxidized oils or oils that may be past their shelf life.

Aromatic medicine educator Mark Webb sug-gests that if citrus oils do not smell like fresh fruit, this means they are oxidizing and one should discontinue use. He goes on to caution not to use them for cleaning or diffusing as you are simply spreading around oxidized oil.

## Skin Reactions

Using proper dilution, following appropriate precautions, and noting age or circumstantial limitations can reduce the risks of using essential oils. However, you do need to know what to look for in the case of an adverse reaction.

*Dermal irritation/toxicity* has degrees: low, medium, or high. Dilution of an essential oil is the only safe way to lessen the chance of all levels of dermal irritation. An oil with low-level dermal irritation means there is a low chance of your skin's reacting to the oil. These oils, such as lavender, are considered the safest for beginners to use. Medium-dermal irritation oils are those that require some moderation in use; dilution is necessary and investigation of precautions should be consulted. High-dermal irritation oils, such as oregano, should never be used undiluted (ever); always consult their precautions for use and dosage.

Reactions can range from redness, rash, itching, and irritation to burning and inflammation of the application site. This is not detoxification; this is your body saying this is not a good match. If a reaction occurs, use straight carrier oils, such as coconut oil, to dilute the essential oil on the skin. Then, you must wash off the area with plenty of soap and water (water alone only spreads the essential oils around further), removing as much of the oil as you can to avoid further irritation.

*Sensitization*, sometimes referred to as hyper-sensitization, is when the body has a response to the particular essential oil, sometimes immediately, sometimes after years of use, and it can appear at random. When sensitization occurs, the particular essential oil can no longer be used—often for years, and possibly permanently. This reaction may come on suddenly after many years of using an oil without any prior problems. It may be triggered by overuse over long term, or by dilutions with more drops of essential oil than appropriate. Think of this as the body has had all it can take and no longer tolerates this relationship in a healthy manner. The response is similar to an allergic reaction.

*Idiosyncratic irritation* is a reaction that is seemingly unusual for a commonly used oil, but for some

## STORY THYME

While learning the distillation process one summer, we distilled clove buds. The aroma was beautifully fragrant: first, the sweet smell of burnt or caramelized sugar, then a cinnamon scent, then a sweet alcohol fragrance, and finally, just as it was dripping hydrosol, the delicious aroma of banana bread or bananas Foster.

As we worked, a few drops would drip on the black metal base that was holding the hydrosol/essential oil receptacle. The oil was so strong, it was peeling the black paint right off!

Consider this a warning: Just because something smells great does not mean it is harmless! Clove is not meant to be used orally. The old remedy for toothaches was meant for the tooth only, not the gums. Do not use on infants!

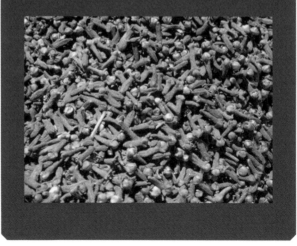

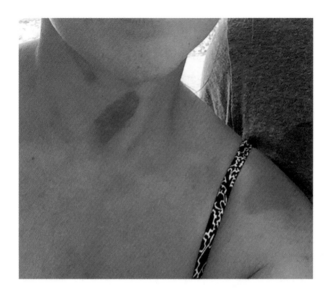

other form of UV light. Dilution is very important, as well as alternative forms of use (such as a personal inhaler) if you will be in the sun, instead of topical application.

## Important Note about Oral Applications of Essential Oils

As noted earlier, oral application or ingestion of essential oils should be avoided, unless suggested by a qualified aromatherapist or a medical doctor trained in aromatherapy. The risk of irritation of the mucous membranes is too high for even small amounts to make contact with the cells. Pain or irritation occurs only after several layers of stomach or esophageal membranes have been affected, and by then, there has been damage.

Essential oils do not mix with water; they remain suspended in the liquid, undiluted, at a high concentration. Therefore, it is not safe to drink water, tea or coffee, or other beverages to which essential oils have been added. I knew a woman who had been advised by a representative of an essential oil company (not a trained aromatherapist) to ingest oregano oil when she felt a cold coming on. She duly added a few drops to a glass of water and drank it down—and experienced throat and digestive troubles immediately, including burning sensations that lasted for weeks afterward. Pure essential oils are not food grade. Food-grade oils (GRAS status) are used in minute dilutions for flavoring, such as in

reason, with this person, the relationship does not match.

*Photosensitization* can occur with certain oils that have the ability to absorb UV light. Your skin can be seriously damaged and you will not feel the effects as they are taking place. While your skin is healing from the burn, it will also show signs of deep pigmentation (different from sunburn). This image here shows a woman who is in the healing phase of having been burned by using undiluted bergamot right before going for a morning run. I am appreciative that her sharing this image may be able to prevent others from going through an accidental and uncomfortable experience. Read each oil's precautions carefully, check the citrus oils chart on page 178, and avoid using photosensitive oils 12 to 24 hours before sun exposure, tanning beds, or any

foods or toothpaste; they are nowhere near the concentrated levels that would cause harm. It is better to consume the plant-based food, tea, or tincture of the source, than the essential oil of a plant.

If you have a real interest in examining using essential oils for internal application, become a certified or clinical aromatherapist first, then train as an aromatic medicine practitioner, learning more about chemistry, botany, herbalism, anatomy, and physiology.

## Neat Application

*Neat* means to apply directly to the skin in small amounts, undiluted. In the past, two oils commonly suggested for neat application were *Lavandula angustifolia* (true lavender) and tea tree. However, overexposure to neat oils, unknowing application of oxidized oils, and sensitization due to overuse can produce adverse skin reactions, allergic responses, and risks of not being able to use an oil ever again. For home use, always use diluted oils unless you have specific instructions from a qualified aromatherapist. Here's a fun reminder: "Salute, Dilute! Keep it sweet, don't use neat."

### MYTH: "THERAPEUTIC GRADE" ESSENTIAL OILS ARE THE BEST.

"Therapeutic grade" is a misnomer because there are no governing bodies that grade essential oils or companies; that is, there aren't any official standards. Marketing companies that suggest their oil is more therapeutic than another company's are using clever wording to get consumers' attention. In fact, essential oils, as pure, unadulterated, nonsynthetic products, are *all* therapeutic in some way. What consumers need to avoid are essential oils that have been adulterated, and synthetic fragrance oils that have no therapeutic value but simply smell (good or bad). If the price is crazy inexpensive, the scent is likely synthetic. Lab-produced chemicals are not going to have the same response physically, mentally, emotionally, or spiritually as the phytocompounds derived from a genuine plant source. If you are looking for essential oils for therapeutic purposes, purchase pure essential oils from a reputable source.

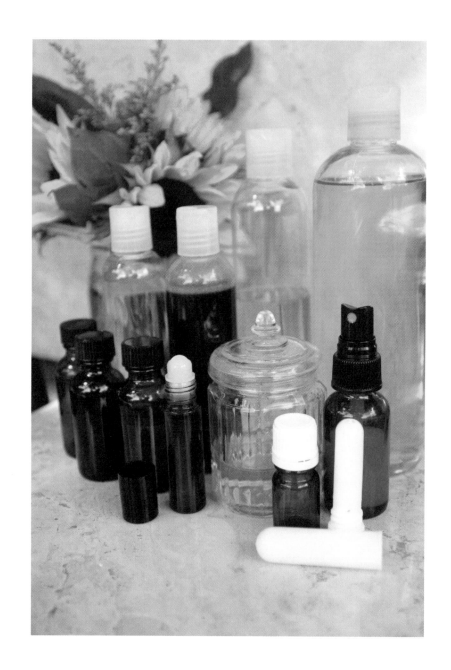

# CHAPTER 6

# Ways to Use Essential Oils

*The little things? The little moments? They aren't little.*
—Jon Kabat-Zinn

Each time you use essential oils, an opportunity to connect with nature as well as your inner being is created. Being mindful of appropriate application of essential oils will help prolong their use and help you discover safe and creative ways to experience your oils. While there are many ways to use essential oils, choose wisely, taking each drop into account for the well-being of your body, mind, and spirit.

## INHALATION

By far, the easiest, and gentlest use of essential oils is simply to enjoy their scent. The aroma given off by the actual plant source is about as pure a resource as you can get—a wonderful way to connect with nature as well as to benefit from its essential oils. Inhaling the scent from a bottled essential oil still connects you to its plant's amazing powers.

There are several ways to do inhalation. The most direct is to open the bottle and take a few breaths. This chapter describes wonderful ways to introduce essential oils to your body, mind, and spirit.

Placing a few drops on an organic cotton ball, paper towel or tissue, or sheet of watercolor paper can be a nice way of following the changes an essential oil goes through in a 24-hour period. Gently waft it under your nose every other hour and see what you notice!

Personal inhalers, aromawands, and aromasticks allow for personal blends in a travel-size container, can hold from 15 to 30 drops of essential oil, last for several months, and are great for school age children and above.

Palm inhalation is a method of dropping a few drops onto your bare hands, rubbing them together, then bringing your palms 4 to 6 inches away from your nose (keep your eyes closed to protect them from the vapors) and inhaling deeply to assist with mind, emotions, and sinus issues. This particular use is generally done with neat (direct) application. Not all oils are appropriate for palm inhalation, so limit this use until you learn more about the individual essential oils.

## DIFFUSERS

Diffusers come in several forms. The easiest to use and the most widely available on the commercial market are water diffusers. These have a small container that usually holds about ⅓ cup of water; you add the essential oils directly to the water. Close the lid (usually a PET plastic lid or ceramic cover, or both), turn on the device, and it will vaporize the water, carrying the essential oils into the air.

Running a diffuser in a room or building with a closed ventilation system means that everyone who is in the area breathes in the essential oils, which may not be desirable by all. Another caution has

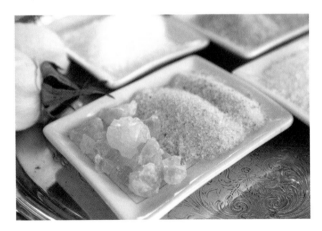

to do with long-term exposure. To prevent triggering sensitization to an oil (see page 97), enjoy your diffuser for 30 minutes, then turn it off for an hour or two. You can enjoy it several times a day, but do so intermittently. Also, change up the oils you are using, to give your body a break. Turn off all diffusers at night to avoid overexposure, blood saturation, and sensitization. For these same reasons, diffusing in classrooms, day care centers, public gathering areas, and offices should be avoided (there's no way to know everyone's health concerns, allergy risks, or respiratory sensitivities).

To keep your water diffuser clean, dispose of any unused water at the end of the day and wipe with a clean cloth or paper towel to prevent bacteria, which can build up quickly (within 48 hours). I have heard of people who use the same water for a week! That is not a good idea because of the potential of bacteria being misted into the air—just because it smells good does not mean it is clean.

Other diffusers on the market are atomizers (no water is used—a fine mist of pure essential oil molecules therefore stay in the air longer) and candle diffusers (which use tea lights under ceramic bowls that hold a bit of water and essential oil).

## ROOM SPRITZERS

An easy way to freshen a room is to put a few drops of essential oils in a PET plastic or glass spray bottle of water or alcohol. Shake vigorously before spraying; a few mists into the air should be

## BATHE SAFELY

Dropping essential oils into running bath water and hopping in has created some surprising, uncomfortable, and intense reactions from skin and mucous membranes! Sensitive regions of the groin, broken skin, and the tender skin of small children may have a faster than expected response to essential oil contact. Adults have reported such reactions as hot/cold, tingling, burning, or freezing sensations in the entire groin area, including reproductive and urinary tract openings, due to the extreme concentration of essential oils. Skin irritations and harmful dermal toxic reactions have also been reported. Be safe, *always dilute* properly, and add to the bath only after getting into the water. And *never* put essential oils straight into a child's bath, no matter how good your intentions are. Do not allow young children to add essential oils to the bath by themselves. Always supervise (and dilute).

sufficient. Because water and oil do not truly mix, do not spray onto wood or delicate fabrics, such as silk. If you would like to explore a better dispersal, try adding a bit of dispersant to your spritzer solution. (One dispersant is Solubol, which can be ordered online, and which can also be used in baths and water-based blends.) Water-based sprays need to be used or discarded within a few days to avoid bacteria and fungus (which can form before you can see/smell it!). Linen/room sprays in an alcohol base (preferably 190 proof) will be self-preserving, lasting until the mixture is used up.

The best way to create a refreshing (and safer) room mist is to skip the essential oils and use hydrosols (see page 230). Hydrosols are gentle, safe enough for contact on skin. Jade Shutes, cofounder of the New York Institute of Aromatic Studies, used lavender hydrosols as a gentle "lavender rain" mist when she tucked her son into bed at night. This little ritual introduced the scent and lavender's benefits into the air without the need for a diffuser. Her son learned to associate the smell of lavender with the pleasant experience and, by extension, with relaxation. Rose or neroli hydrosol is another bedtime room mist you can use with children (or teens/adults!). Hydrosols are also fantastic for calming active children during playtime, or when signs of overstimulation are present.

The water in diffusers can also be replaced by hydrosols for an added benefit to your blend. Hydrosols used in room spritzers or diffusers are recommended for children, the elderly, and those in fragile conditions. Hydrosols also make great toners on a clean face before moisturizing.

## BATHS
Hydrotherapy is a valuable and long tradition in the healing arts. Bathhouses were used for social and health reasons thousands of years

ago, and they are still used in some areas around the world. Soaking in a warm bath with essential oils has been recommended over the last several decades, but the application has not been clarified for the general public to do safely at home. Please *do not* just drop essential oils in a warm bath and climb in. Water and oil do not mix. Essential oil will sit on the water's surface if you sprinkle in the oil while the tub is filling. Even if you swish the water around, the oil will resettle on the surface. When you step in, the straight essential oil touches your body first and could be very damaging (see sidebar "Bathe Safely," page 103).

Instead, disperse a few drops of essential oil in any of the following: 2% or full-fat milk; cream; or emulsified soaps, such as liquid body wash, shampoo, or even bubble bath. The fatty substance and the oil-based product will recognize each other and blend themselves in a diluted solution. Get into the warm bath *first* and *then* add the mixture to the bath. Epsom salts, in place of the milk/soap base, is acceptable for low dermal toxic oils. These methods are safe for all ages in appropriate dilutions per age groups. Additionally, add a carrier oil with your essential oils first before mixing with salt, especially with any mixtures that have any precautions of skin irritation.

Here is an easy way to create bath salts: Mix 1 teaspoon of carrier oil, such as coconut, jojoba, or sweet almond, with 5 drops of an essential oil, such as lavender, or of an essential oil synergy (use only low dermal irritant blends and oils). Add this mixture to 1 cup of salt (Epsom salts, Himalayan pink salt, Dead Sea salt, sea salt, or a combination) in a lidded glass or nonreactive metal container. Alternatively, to ensure proper safe use, add a dispersant, such as Solubol. Mix thoroughly. Seal and leave for at least 24 hours.

This amount will be suitable for one or two baths, depending on how much you would like to use. Add the salts to a bath and swish it around while the tub is being filled. Enjoy for 15 to 20 minutes.

You may use the same procedure for a wonderful foot bath, hand soak, or sitz bath, reducing the salt and essential oils by half.

## MASSAGE

You do not have to be a massage therapist to enjoy the benefits of massaging your own body and that of others. Infant massage was introduced in the hospital

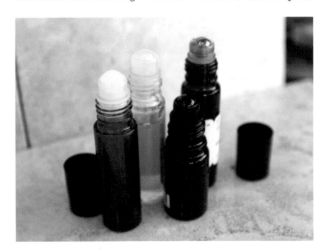

to Liz Fulcher after she gave birth to her child when she was living in France. The gentle touch, helping her baby feel calm and loved, using a wonderfully gentle carrier, was how she began her introduction to aromatherapy . . . which ended up blossoming into her business as an aromatherapy educator and founder of the Aromatic Wisdom Institute. Children love a goodnight back rub or foot massage. Even a gentle hand massage is wonderful at bedtime for children (as long as they are old enough to not put their hand in their mouth after a massage). Carriers alone are best for babies; no essential oils are needed.

Ayurveda supports self-massage called *abhyanga*, using warm oil to rejuvenate the mind and body. Doing self-massage every day (perfect for right before bed or just out of the shower) aids in moving lymph, increases blood circulation, supports digestion with abdominal massage, relaxes the mind and emotions, and opens the spirit.

Don't have time to give yourself a full body massage every day? Many people do not. However, doing small massage movements can have exponential benefits. Consider blending a few nice oils, such as lavender, mandarin, rose geranium, or clary sage, in an unscented lotion and massaging your clean feet before you go to bed. (Run any leftover residue from your fingers through your hair to add a nice wisp of scent as you sleep.)

Slow massage movements are best for relaxation (and sore muscles!); light movements are the most supportive for lymph; and vigorous strokes are for increasing circulation in an area.

## BLENDS

A blend can be any combination of essential oils within a carrier oil, lotion, cream, gel, or bath salt. In Chapters 15, 16, and 17 of this book (as well as bonus recipes in the essential oils profiles), you will learn how to create your own blends for different uses.

Lotions and creams are great for massage, feet, and hands.

Gels are best for fungal issues and cooling inflammatory skin concerns, such as sunburn.

Carrier oils are wonderful for hair and skin (but not necessarily for the bottoms of the feet or palms of hands; use lotions and creams instead). Do not use carrier oils on fungus; use gel-based products or compresses instead.

Master blends, a.k.a. synergies, can be mixed ahead and diluted or diffused later. For instance, if I really loved the combination of sweet orange, patchouli, and ylang-ylang to reduce stress and tension during my personal yoga practice at home, I could mix the correct number of drops for a synergy in a 5 ml amber or cobalt blue glass bottle. Then, it would be ready in the right proportions in this one bottle, to add two or three drops to my diffuser at yoga time.

## ROLLER BALLS

Placing a small amount of essential oils, generally five or six drops total, in a 10 ml bottle topped with a metal or plastic PET roller ball creates an easy-to-use, travel-ready, handy means of using essential oils as a personal perfume or for spot

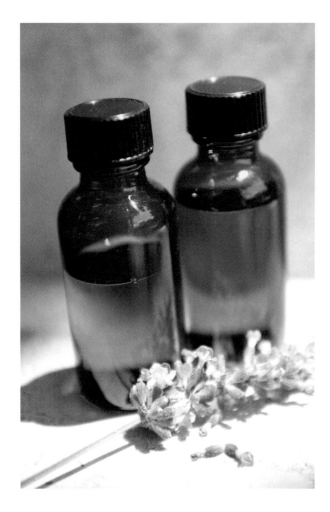

and keep the dilution to the appropriate age (see Chapter 15). Anything used on the face needs to be highly diluted, no more than 1.5% total, with no more than four drops maximum in a 10 ml bottle. Acne spot treatments can have up to 5% dilution, but should not be applied all over the face, only to the specific area, hence the "spot" in "spot application."

Roller balls can be great introductions to teaching self-care to teens, children, and those who are new to taking care of themselves. As roller balls are for minimal applications, 10 ml bottles are the perfect size.

If the carrier of your choice begins to smell bad, your blend has oxidized and you must discontinue use. Do not use on your skin, as you increase the risk of dermal sensitivity. If at any time your skin shows signs of irritation, rash, or itchiness, stop use, as your blend may be oxidizing, and discard the blend.

## STEAM INHALATION

Steam inhalation is helpful for congestion and sinus stuffiness. Conifer oils, such as pine, fir, and spruce, plus the eucalyptus species, work great with respiratory issues. Lavender, palmarosa, patchouli, rose geranium, and clary sage are nice facial steam essential oils.

Heating water hot enough to create a bit of steam (not to a boil) is all that is needed to open the pores of the skin and deliver a warm hydrated mist of essential oils to the skin, sinuses, and

applications. (Do not apply by this method all over the body or face.) Keep your dilutions appropriate for the application. If you are creating a blend for bug bites for children, you will need to use child-appropriate essential oils, such as lavender,

respiratory system along with beneficial mood-enhancing effects. Add three to five drops of an essential oil to the warm water (be careful; the pot or bowl may be very hot). Keep your eyes closed to protect them from the oils in the steam, lean over, and drape a towel over your head (for children, omit using a towel to reduce any risk of burning the skin or sinus cavities). Hold this position for 5 to 15 minutes.

## COMPRESS, HOT AND COLD

Hot and warm compresses are very soothing for sore muscles and congested chest colds. Pour warm water into a glass or ceramic bowl (do not use metal, wooden, or plastic bowls). You will want the water as hot as can safely be handled; do not use scalding or boiling water. Add a few drops of essential oil (conifers and eucalyptus species do well for respiratory support) and swish around. For more safely dispersed dilutions, add essential oils to salt with a very small amount of carrier oil, let them absorb, then add the scented salt to the water and let it all dissolve, creating a therapeutic saline solution. (A cup of water, ¼ teaspoon of salt, ⅛ to ¼ teaspoon of carrier oil and one or two drops of essential oil should be fine.) Quickly drench a small towel in the hot mixture, then ring it out so no liquid is dripping. Place the towel on the sore muscle, back, or chest. You can cover the towel with a second, dry towel to soak up any dripping water and to keep the heat in for a few minutes longer. Change out the towel in 15 minutes.

Warm compresses are wonderful muscle soothers for menstrual cramps (try Roman chamomile and clary sage). Essential oils such as cardamom, fennel, and Roman chamomile are helpful in a compress for an upset stomach.

Cool compresses are best suited for inflammation or fevers. With the same method, only using cool water, add anti-inflammatory essential oils, such as low dilutions of lavender, Roman chamomile, or rosalina (using hydrosols with this method works well for children).

Do not put compresses that contain essential oils over the eyes. Instead, wet a clean towel with plain water or substitute hydrosols. Hydrosols are great for children, teens, and adults.

Use low dermal irritant essential oils in low dilutions for compresses (keeping in mind that water and oil will not fully disperse on their own).

## Final Notes for Using Essential Oils

Here are a few simple guidelines to keep in mind when using essential oils.

### START WITH THREE OILS

You do not need to have an entire kit to gain a ton of benefit from essential oils. Pick three oils that have some variety in use and aroma. I suggest a flower, a conifer or citrus, and either an earthy or a woody oil, to start. With these three you will have plenty to touch on the emotional gentleness of a floral note; the conifer or citrus can lighten up the energy of the room and brighten the spirit; an earthy or woody aroma will act as a grounded note when finding your center is important. Whichever oils you choose, learn about them, feel them, and open yourself to the relationship between you and these oils.

### USE OFTEN, AS NEEDED, BUT NOT NECESSARILY EVERY DAY

Essential oils are concentrated. As overusing can create systemic complications, use your oils lightly and only as needed. Keep in mind that your body is amazing and should not ordinarily require essential oils; keep them for when it does. Plus, you help the planet replenish its resources with mindful usage. Obtaining new oils without purpose can be wasteful, as the plants take time to grow to the maturity level of essential oil harvest.

Essential oils are not *preventative* as much as they are *active*. They actively create change in mind, body, and emotions upon release. Use the oils with direct intention and purpose to prevent wasting these precious gems and avoid overload on the body.

### ROTATE YOUR OILS

Using a variety of oils helps rotate your shelf stock as well as gives your body a break from overexposure to the same oils. Plus, switching them up will help strengthen your sense of smell and the connection that each oil has with your body. As you rotate your oils, your ability to be aware of the benefits of an essential oil will increase with use, time, and patience.

### ASK QUESTIONS

If you are not sure about what an oil can do, look it up; don't guess or rely on fuzzy memory. *Always learn about an essential oil before using it*—and read about it again (especially for cautions or contraindications) if you haven't used it in a while. For example, I love the scent of fennel (especially mixed with sweet orange and a dash of laurel in a diffuser), but that does not mean it is safe for everyone; for instance, it should be avoided in all forms during pregnancy and breastfeeding.

Do pay attention to your sources of information. There is an abundance of "free advice" on social media and other Internet sites. If you are unsure, cross-check details with a reputable source that has been properly trained in the field of aromatherapy (not just someone who sells essential oils).

Okay—are you ready to meet some new friends? You have heard so much about them! Let's introduce you to the essential oils.

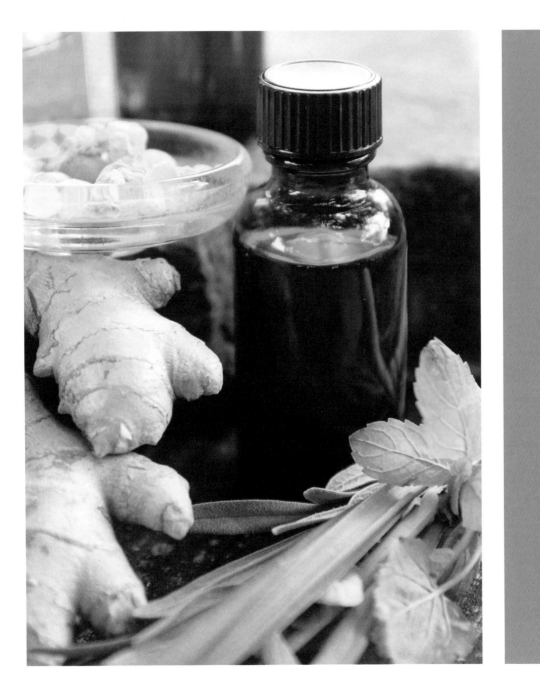

# Aromatics

**3**

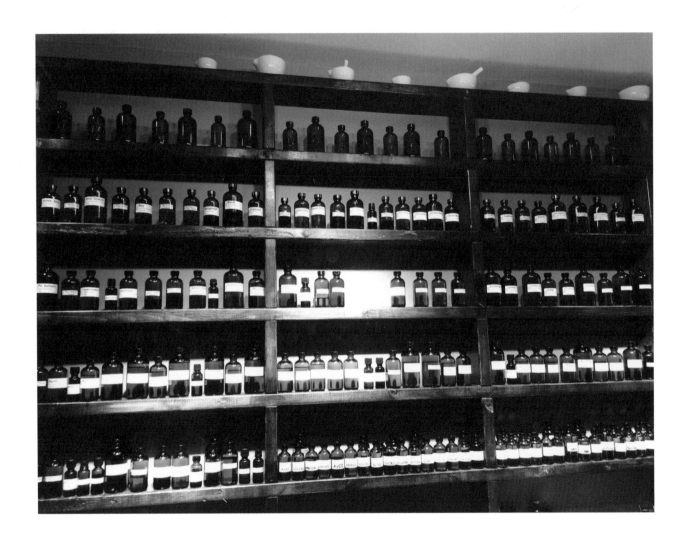

# CHAPTER 7

# Essential Oils to Have in Your Home

**You do not need every oil discussed here.** It is fine to begin with just a few and then add more from there (it can be helpful to have a few options according to your needs). But please read this first before proceeding to the individual oils.

## Allow an Introduction

When many people first open a bottle of oil, they take a big sniff and decide immediately whether they like it or not. But remember, an oil is an accumulation of ancient wisdom within the plant as well as a concentrated version of that plant's protective and attractive properties. You need to engage your senses more fully from the start:

1. Feel: Hold the bottle, cap closed, for a moment and be still. Very sensitive people can feel the vibration of the essence of the oil as it connects with them simply by holding it. Others may not feel anything at first, and that's okay. But if you are sensitive, it is important to trust even the smallest responses of your body.

2. Smell: Open the bottle and hold it down by your waist, the core of your body, with your eyes closed if possible, rather than near your nose. See whether you can smell the oil from there. Slowly move the bottle upward and notice when you first begin to smell the aroma as it approaches your nose. This exercise can help you understand the potency of how "big" an aroma is with a certain oil. Let the aroma find its way to you. A secondary exercise is to wave just the cap, beneath your nose, which may sometimes share deeper notes than the lovely top notes that first leave a bottle.

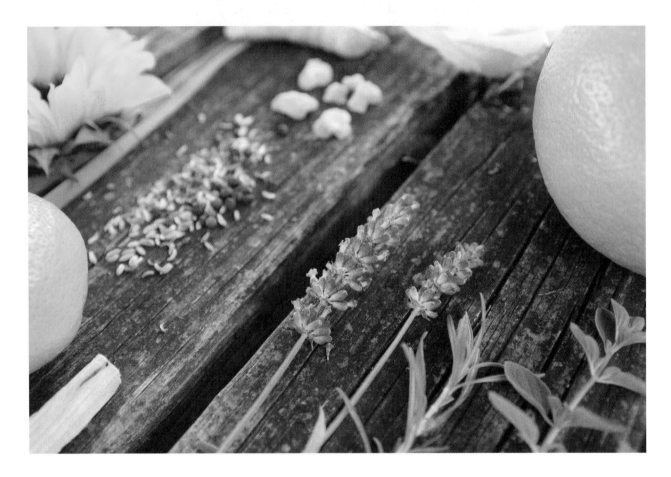

3. Taste: Inhale with your mouth slightly open, to allow your taste buds to participate. (*Caution: This is about breathing; do not put the essential oil in your mouth!*) They have systematic responses that can help you smell better, the same way your sense of smell can help foods taste better. Some oils, especially those that help support digestion, may stimulate your taste buds. For example, you might notice your saliva production increases just by your smelling a warm, spicy oil. You might also notice right away that smelling an adulterated or synthetic oil will leave a chemical taste in your mouth.

4. Notice: What is the initial response your body or mind has to the oil? Do you find you want to

breathe deeper? Does it remind you of something or is it new and unfamiliar? Do you immediately start to relax? Does your brain begin to focus better? Does a deeper part of yourself begin to feel more connected? It's okay if you don't notice anything at first. It takes training for you to become aware of the ways you respond to an oil. I call these "indicators." With awareness and practice, you will learn to trust your indicators.

5. Invite: Sensory experiences are more than physical. Exchanging the wisdom from an aromatic plant through its essential oil is very much like developing a relationship. Inviting a new experience, allowing the oil to share its character and personality, may open observation in a whole new way. Some people develop a resonance with certain essential oils by simply inviting the exchange to be deeper than superficial. For instance, smelling a base note oil can give the impression of a low, deep drum vibrating through the body or lying on the earth totally supported head to toe. Each experience will be unique and individual. It might be as simple as "there is something about this oil I really like."

In the world of essential oils, you will find descriptions go far beyond "It smells like a flower." The following guide lists ways that aromatherapists describe certain oils. See whether these words help

## FRAGRANCE, SCENT, AND ODOR GUIDE

| | |
|---|---|
| Aromatic | Powdery |
| Balsamic | Powerful |
| Bitter | Pungent |
| Bittersweet | Radiant |
| Camphoraceous | Rancid |
| Citrusy | Refreshing |
| Clean | Resinous |
| Cool | Rich |
| Earthy | Rootlike |
| Fecal | Rosy |
| Fiery | Sharp |
| Floral | Smoky |
| Fresh | Soft |
| Fruity | Spicy-sweet |
| Grassy | Tenacious |
| Green | Terpenic |
| Haylike | Uplifting |
| Heavy | Vannilic |
| Herbaceous | Warm |
| Honey-scented | Woody |
| Hot | Zesty |
| Intense | |
| Leafy-woody | |
| Light | |
| Medicinal | |
| Mild | |
| Musky | |
| Nutty | |
| Penetrating | |
| Peppery | |

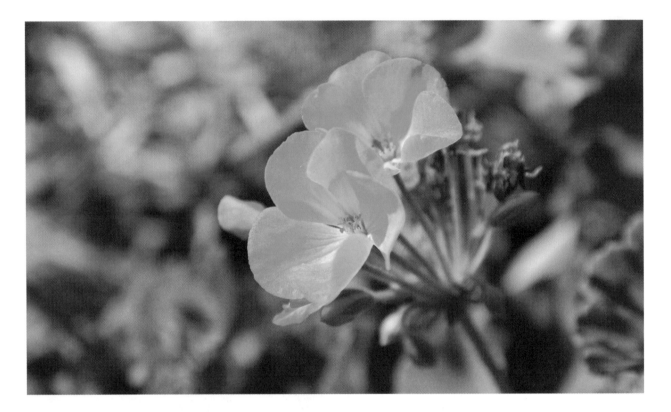

you identify aromas as you begin to explore essential oils for yourself. It will help train and strengthen your sense of smell, too!

Many brands of essential oils are available from reputable sources that are direct distributors from distillers. Keep it simple for yourself.

- Always refer to the Safety Guide (page 92) and Chapters 5 and 6.
- Ask questions: Where does a distributer obtain its oils? Does it use online resources or have an established relationship with a distiller? Where did the oil come from? (Oils' aroma may vary, due to differences relating to location or harvesting/distillation.)
- Use multiple sources, if necessary, rather than being married to one brand. Support the industry and your health at the same time.
- Be mindful of the differences between species within a genus; read the properties and purpose of each essential oil.
- Seek good-quality carriers and dilute properly

(see Chapters 15 and 16), and be aware of any cautions or contraindications.

- Avoid outdated, oxidized, and synthetic oils as well as "fragrance" oils (not the same as natural perfume).
- Each oil has distinctive properties, so before using, read about and learn to distinguish among the many oils. Unless suggested to do so, do not simply substitute one for another.
- If you already have some essential oils, I highly recommend smelling them while you further research them, to help you identify their observable components as you read.
- Beyond all practical suggestions, learning about and being open to the subtleties available through essential oils is just as important.

## The Essential Oils

Like a Venn diagram, all essential oils innately have overlapping qualities as well as areas of uniqueness. In some cases, there is also overlap in which part of the plant is used. The essential oils are arranged in categories according to the part of the plant from which they are associated. For instance, I have placed rosemary in the category of stems, leaves, and needles, but its flowers can also be included in distillation, and so also reading about petals and flowers would be helpful. Normally placed within the category of berries, I have placed black pepper with

**STORY THYME**

Getting to know essential oils is a lot like discovering music.

At first, you might like a song you hear on the radio, then begin to recognize the lead singer's voice in other songs, then the band's distinctive sound. Soon you know more about the members of the band, and share their music with others.

Essential oils are a little like hearing that song on the radio. First, you like a scent, learn its name and character, and begin to identify it within a blend, and then you share its qualities with others.

It is easy to fall in love with the individual voices of essential oils and it is quite amazing to become part of their song.

seeds as the amount of fruit is minuscule compared to the size of the seed in the harvested plant material (but do note that the entire fruit is technically harvested, then dried). You may also think of these groupings as reflecting plants' stages of development, to help you associate some of their character traits.

These wonderful oils will get you started on a wide range of single notes you can use individually or to make your own blends for personal and home use. Enjoy!

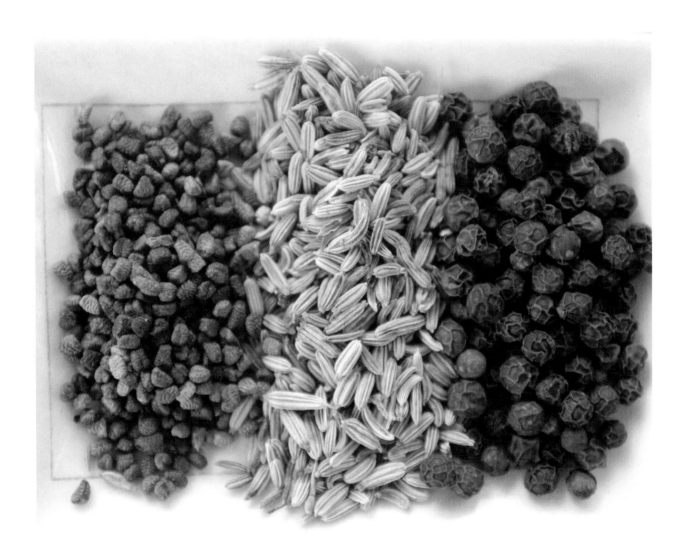

# CHAPTER 8

# Seeds

*You were designed for accomplishment, engineered for success, and endowed with the seeds of greatness.* —Zig Ziglar

## Potential—Awaken—Ignite

Seeds (and nuts) are pure potential, containing the matrix, or blueprint, of an entire plant, bringing with them the wisdom and perseverance of the deepest, inner nature of their original plant, the mother, upon release. Seeds' job is to go out into the world and create new life. Once a seed has found the place to grow, the alchemic shift of roots going deep down into the earth and the seedling's breaking ground above the surface shift the energy from a single solid mass into a dynamic force of further possibility. Conversely, seeds' protective outer layer shield their inner blueprint, which lies dormant until conditions are right for action to occur.

Seeds and nuts are the source of many carrier oils.

## Cardamom

*Warmth—Appetite—Harmony*
**Common name:** Cardamom
**Latin name:** *Ellettaria cardomomum*
**Botanical family:** Zingiberaceae; relatives are ginger and turmeric.

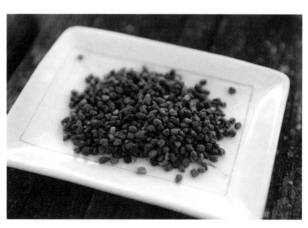

**Attributes:** When combined with other oils in small doses, cozy, warm, friendly, and gently stimulating. Some people love cardamom immediately; others warm up to it a little at a time.

**Character:** A tall, erect, leafy perennial, grown from rhizome, which can reach up to 9 feet in height. Likes tropical, humid environments with just the right amount of sun. The flowers are usually white with a dash of yellow, red, or violet in stripes from the center outward. When the blooms dry out, they transform into a fruit pod called a capsule. It takes up to three years of growth to produce the mature capsules containing seeds.

Cardamom's most common use is as a spice; also, the seeds have been used in Chinese and Ayurvedic medicines for more than three millennia. Its essential oil is a bit warming and requires some care when used. It may cost a bit more than other essential oils.

**Unique aroma:** Warm, sweet, woody, floral undertones, balsamic, spicy

**Aromatic note:** Mid to base

**Part of plant used for essential oils:** Seed

**Countries of origin:** Primarily India; also Guatemala and Sri Lanka

**Actions:** Antibacterial, antifungal, antispasmodic, aphrodisiac, digestive stimulant, expectorant, soothes/calms nervous system, stimulant, tonic

**Uses:**

- *Physically:* Breaks up congested airways and sinuses; eases coughs. Try blending with lavender, cedarwood, and sandalwood for a

## Sacred Calm and Uplift

Combine in a water-based room diffuser:

1 drop cardamom

1 drop palo santo

3 drops sweet orange

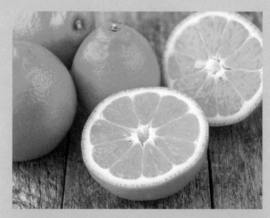

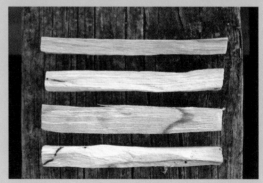

respiratory aid. Cardamom's warm, energetic influences stimulate the digestion system and relieves nausea. Blended with a carrier oil and applied as a massage oil, soothes sore muscles, including menstrual cramps, by stimulating peripheral circulation and relieving pain. Aids digestion when blended with black pepper, ginger, fennel, and sweet orange in a muscle rub or abdominal massage. Also used in aphrodisiac blends.

- *Mentally:* Acts both as tonic for nervous exhaustion due to overthinking and to bring gentle focus in times of deficient concentration. One drop, along with sweet orange, in a room diffuser can make the room feel a little lighter.
- *Emotionally:* Can calm worry and scattered attention, the feeling that there is not enough of you to go around. Helps the emotional heart feel acknowledged, warmed, and satiated. Also, along with lavender and frankincense, can soothe a distressed emotional heart.
- *Spiritually:* Opens the spirit to uplifting spaces, to proceed with confidence beyond temporary disturbances. Combine with a sacred wood, such as palo santo, for a wonderful meditative synergy or sacred space scent.

**Blends well with:** Bergamot, black pepper, cedarwood, clary sage, fennel, frankincense, ginger, jasmine, lavender, mandarin, palmarosa, palo santo, rose geranium, rose, sandalwood, sweet orange, ylang-ylang

**Precautions:** Generally nonirritating as an aroma. For skin application, always dilute in a carrier; using too much may produce contact dermatitis. Do not use during pregnancy, with infants and small children, or during breastfeeding.

**Shelf life:** 4 to 5 years

# Black Pepper
*Stimulating—Warming—Ancient*

**Common name:** Black pepper

**Latin name:** *Piper nigrum*

**Botanical family:** Piperaceae, which has 2,000 species and five different genera, ranging from climbing vines to shrubs to trees. *P. nigrum* is the only member of the Piperaceae family used for essential oil.

**Attributes:** Stimulating, igniting, fiery, pain relieving, underestimated. Warm and friendly when treated with respect, voted most likely to be the surprise guest in a blend.

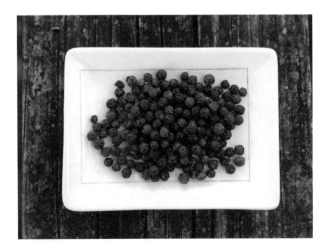

**Character:** As an aromatic perennial, produces flowers and climbs upward toward the sky, thick and vinelike, to a towering height of 20 feet. Happiest in humid, tropical rain forests; takes a couple of years to flourish completely. Pepper berries grow in clusters known as drupes. The spike of the plant (bearing the berries) is picked when an unripe green color. Each dried berry contains a single seed. As the amount of fruit actually contained by these berries is so low, and the seeds remain intact inside them when they are dried, this spice is classed as a seed in this book, showcasing its most predominate component; you will find it as a berry in cross-referencing. While drying, its color transitions from green to red to black; the latter is known as a black peppercorn, long used as a culinary spice. Pepper is historically one of the most widely traded aromatics, recorded as far back as 4,000 years, with uses ranging from Egyptian mummification processes to being demanded as ransom for Rome by Attila the Hun. Once considered an antidote to poison and a remedy for fever.

**Unique aroma:** Warm, sharp, spicy, fresh, woody, peppery, pungent; some noses will detect a clove or floral scent.

**Aromatic note:** Mid

**Part of plant used for essential oils:** Seed (berry)

**Countries of origin:** Indonesia, Malaysia, Madagascar, China, and India

**Actions:** Analgesic, antiseptic, antispasmodic, antitoxic, aphrodisiac, digestive, circulatory tonic, reduces fever, reduces pain (muscles), rubefacient, stimulating

**Uses:**

- *Physically:* Supports the musculoskeletal system well by stimulating peripheral circulation and relieves joint and muscle pain. Can be used to warm up cold muscles prior to strenuous activity. Try blending with ginger, rosemary, lavender, or geranium as a massage oil for muscles. Stimulates digestion (both peristaltic movement and urination) and soothes menstrual discomfort. Works well with fennel, peppermint, cardamom, and ginger for a nice abdominal massage to ease digestive issues. As a respiratory stimulant, encourages expectoration and decongestion, and is a good addition to cold and flu blends, such as eucalyptus, rosemary, and frankincense. Provides energy redirection when there is fatigue. Also acts as a tonic to the circulatory system and a rubefacient.

Rubefacients increase circulation to a localized area, bringing in new blood, which will create a nice warming to the skin and muscles and more redness/pinkness to the skin. This is very different than dermal toxicity, an inflammatory response sometimes accompanied by blotches, a feeling of hot heat, rash, itchiness, general uncomfortableness, or an allergic reaction. If you know your essential oil's properties, you will discern its natural desired effects versus an adverse response.

# Warm My Toes
## (lotion or cream)

In a 1-ounce glass or PET plastic container, create a synergy with the following essential oils *first*, then add 1 ounce of unscented lotion or cream (it mixes best if you add a little lotion at a time instead of all at once). Best for cold toes or in the wintertime; massage, then cover with socks.

10 drops black pepper
5 drops cardamom
5 drops ginger
5 drops fennel

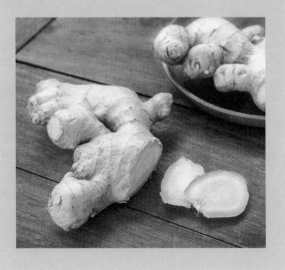

- *Mentally:* Both stimulates the circulation of fresh blood throughout the body and brain, and assists circulation of thoughts by encouraging mental alertness and boosting stamina. Add to a blend with ginger and rosemary to increase mental readiness.
- *Emotionally:* In times of low confidence, an inability to set healthy boundaries, apathy, emotional coldness, mental and emotional fatigue, fragile nerves, anxiety, or insomnia due to emotional depletion, use to ignite the inner resources of the body to reach harmony (also helpful for frigidity). Amazing when blended in a diffuser with sweet orange, mandarin, grapefruit, or bergamot.
- *Spiritually:* Will light the fire within from your inner core outward to the periphery of all the places in your life. Also may increase relaxation, as well as banish negative thinking and clear your thoughts. Add to bring a little warmth to a blend of ginger, palo santo, frankincense, sandalwood, or rose when creating a connection to your spirit.

**Blends well with:** Cardamom, clary sage, clove, fennel, frankincense, geranium, ginger, grapefruit, laurel, lavender, lemon, neroli, palo santo, rose, rosemary, sandalwood, sweet marjoram, tea tree

**Precautions:** Best stored in the refrigerator, as it can create dermal toxic reactions if it oxidizes or goes beyond its shelf life. Do not use old black pepper oil!

**Shelf life:** 3 years

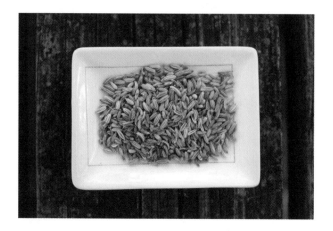

# Sweet Fennel

*Soothing—Digestion—Courage*

**Common names:** Sweet fennel, fennel, fenkel

**Latin name:** *Foeniculum vulgare* var. *dulce*

**Botanical family:** Apiaceae, sometimes known as Umbelliferae, one of the largest flowering aromatic herb families in the plant world and the first flowering family to be named by botanists. Cousins include carrot, celery, dill, and parsley.

**Attributes:** A digestive helper, physically but also emotional and mental digestion. Has a unique connection with women—either serves as a close friend or needs to be avoided. Soothing, warm, quite comforting.

**Character:** A tall perennial, growing from 4 to 6 feet in height, with beautiful light, feathery leaves. In summer, if not harvested, produces tiny yellow flowers at the tips of long umbels. Fennel's main bulb, a root stock, and its seeds are edible.

The seeds are actually tiny fruits, but due to their size and appearance, most people call them seeds. Has been used in Ayurvedic medicine as well as Traditional Chinese Medicine. While another essential oil is made from bitter fennel (*F. vulgare Mill.* spp. *Capillaceum Gilb*), sweet fennel (as indicated in its Latin term *dulce*) is what you need to look for. If in doubt, check the Latin name!

**Unique aroma:** Licorice, sweet, dried grass, haylike, herbaceous, warm, anise, green

**Aromatic note:** Top to mid

**Part of plant used for essential oils:** Seed

**Countries of origin:** Spain, France, Italy, Greece, Turkey, Bulgaria, India, and Japan as well as North America. Considered indigenous to the Mediterranean.

**Special chemical properties:** Particularly high in trans-anethole, which creates a strong contraindication (see Precautions).

**Actions:** Anti-inflammatory, antibacterial, antifungal, antispasmodic, detoxifier, digestive, relieves gas

**Uses:**

- *Physically:* In general, sweet fennel gets the stuck get unstuck. Well known for relieving nausea, bloating, flatulence, and other forms of indigestion. Use in massage or compress is best for this application. Can be combined with cardamom, peppermint, and ginger and massaged on the abdomen. Also dispels coughs and nervous asthma, paired with either eucalyptus or lemon. Stimulates lymphatic movement and sluggish

# Women's Abdominal Massage Blend

*(Adapted from David Crow's Women's Menstrual Blend)*

In a 1-ounce glass bottle, combine the following essential oils, according to proper blending protocols, then add your choice of carrier oil. Close the cap and gently roll, tipping the bottle upside down, then upright, several times. Open and breathe in the scent before massaging in a clockwise motion on the lower abdomen.

2 drops fennel
2 drops clary sage
2 drops rose geranium
2 drops bergamot
2 drops neroli

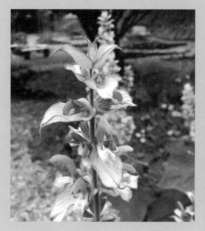 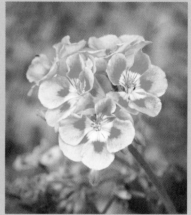

skin (cellulite) when blended with a little black pepper and sweet marjoram. Can relieve menstrual cramps and discomfort by mixing with geranium and clary sage.

- *Mentally:* Sweet fennel's airy physical structure corresponds to its providing lightness of mental and emotional support. It dispels stuck thoughts, especially for those who tend to overthink and need a direction to let go and focus. Used in Ayurveda, helps the mind digest ideas as well as food.

- *Emotionally:* "As above, so below": if your digestive system is slow or blocked, your emotions can often reflect the same drag. Releasing trapped emotions similarly provides confidence. Sweet fennel helps you feel good about yourself by allowing you to better digest your experiences. Combine with sweet orange and laurel in a diffuser for a light, expansive, sweet pick-me-up.

- *Spiritually:* Add a drop to a blend of frankincense, palo santo, vetiver, or patchouli for a grounded lightness in your spiritual practices.

**Blends well with:** Bergamot, cardamom, cinnamon leaf, clary sage, cypress, ginger, grapefruit, lime, mandarin, patchouli, rose geranium, rose, sandalwood, sweet marjoram, sweet orange, ylang-ylang

**Precautions:** Do not use this oil in any manner (diffuser, topical, internal) during pregnancy or breastfeeding, or with children under age 5. Do not use with endometriosis and estrogen dependent cancers. Additionally, may inhibit blood clotting or cause reproduction hormone modulation. Use a maximum of 1.0 to 2.5% in a final dilution for safe dilution (always start at the lowest dilution for your blend). May cause skin reactions if oxidized or improperly diluted.

**Shelf life:** 2 to 4 years

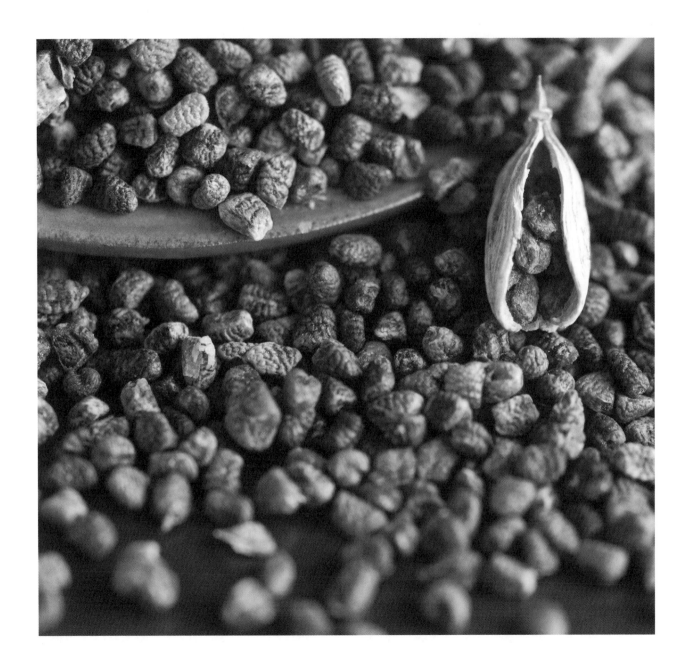

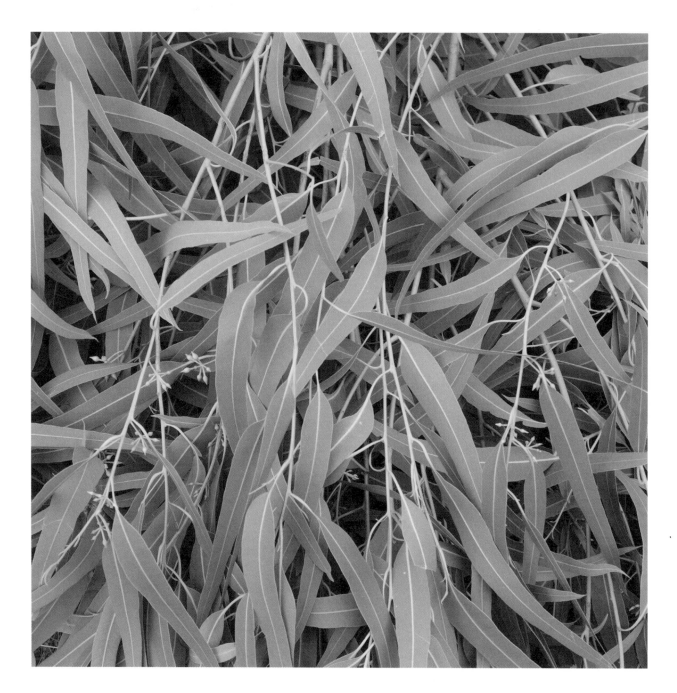

# CHAPTER 9

# Stems, Leaves, and Needles

*Every particular in nature, a leaf, a drop, a crystal, a moment of time
is related to the whole, and partakes of the perfection of the whole.*
—Ralph Waldo Emerson

## Expansion—Breath—Transition

Stems support reaching out and letting go with the support of an internal anchor. Leaves and needles are opening and expanding, inviting the breath of life to exchange in and out.

To be the part of a plant that moves away from its core represents a step of courage, a steady reach into the potential outside the inner base. Branching out allows for expressions of freedom and natural transitions: stems, leaves, and needles sometimes alternate, sometimes align symmetrically as they grow; as such, they are among the important botanical identification markers of a plant. All provide the life-supporting exchange between a species and its outside environment through the sun, the moon, transpiration, respiration, and vaporization.

## Cistus (Rock Rose)

*Antibacterial—Unfurling—Deeply soothing*
**Common names:** Cistus or rock rose
**Latin name:** *Cistus ladaniferus*
**Botanical family:** Cistaceae, small family of shrubs

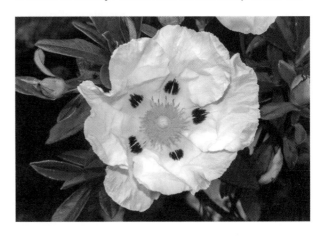

that tends to prefer dry and sunny habitats. There are many varieties of species within this family; you may even find some in your backyard or landscape.

**Attributes:** Mysterious yet comforting and soothing; also an excellent emotional and immunity booster. Good in blends; a little bit goes a long way. Some people are not sure what to think when they first smell this aroma, but cistus is a fascinating oil to add to blends.

**Character:** When in bloom, cistus's papery flowers, colored white with deep burgundy droplets near the yellow center, expand strikingly against the evergreen leaves. The branches tend to open up like an umbrella in all directions, ranging from 3 to 8 feet in width and height. Has been used historically as an aromatic plant in traditional medicines to relieve intestinal pain and diarrhea, and for catarrhal and menstrual discomfort, as well as in incense and perfumes. Its resin was first discovered well before its distilled oil was ever produced. (Historically, the wool of the sheep and hair from goats going through cistus patches has been used to collect the resin, which is then combed out.) Labdanum, a deep base note used in incense and perfumery, comes from its resin and gum. The essential oil, used in perfumes and essential oil blends, ranges in color from deep amber to dark yellow, depending on where the plant is cultivated, and can have a bit of a green hue as well.

**Unique aroma:** Musky, rich, spicy, warm, green, floral, enduring, herbaceous, resinous, a tad earthy, a whisper of sweetness. Cistus reminds me of desert

## Wound-Healing First-Aid Gel Spray
### (safe for children and adults)

In a 2-ounce bottle with a spray top, combine the following:

10 drops lavender

10 drops helichrysum

6 drops frankincense (*Boswellia carteri*)

6 drops Roman chamomile

4 drops cistus

6 drops rosalina

2 tablespoons rose hydrosol

10 to 11 drops Solubol dispersant (optional)

Fill the rest of the container with:

Aloe vera gel (inner fillet)

Shake and spray as needed. Store in the refrigerator. Use within 1 to 2 months. Label properly.

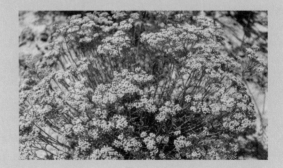

flowers after a deep torrential rain, and other times, conjures up images of being inside a cave with exotic flowering plants.

**Aromatic note:** Base

**Part of plant used for essential oils:** Stems, twigs, and dried leaves (and sometimes dried flowers)

**Countries of origin:** Mediterranean, especially Spain, Portugal, Morocco, France, and Crete; also some areas of North and South America

**Special chemical properties:** Contains more than 250 unique compounds, giving cistus complexity therapeutically and aromatically.

**Actions:** Aids in abating surface bleeding (cictrisant), antibacterial, anti-infectious, antimicrobial, astringent, antiviral, immunity booster and regulator, tonic and support for parasympathetic and central nervous systems, wound healing

**Uses:**

- *Physically:* Known to be quite relaxing as can help regulate the parasympathetic ("rest and rejuvenate") nervous system. Also helps clear respiratory infections. Has been used to brighten aging skin while promoting skin, nail, and hair health, especially in mature skin. Aids in sleep disorders, such as insomnia, and soothes migraines and headaches. Relieves muscular and joint pains as well as discomforts of rheumatism, neuralgia, and carpal tunnel and restless leg syndromes. Benefits damaged tissue, such as cuts and acne. Has been used as a disinfectant for wounds due to its astringent and antibacterial compounds.

- *Mentally:* Clears the way to positive thinking, energizing the psyche and soothing the thought process, while supporting the parasympathetic nervous system.

- *Emotionally:* Entices the mind and emotions to release their hold on old ways, encouraging forward movement. Like the bursting of flowers in spring, can assist in opening and encouragement.

- *Spiritually:* By clearing thoughts, gently sharing possibilities of clear pathways, symbolically removing debris from the skin and healing the wounds of abrasive experiences, and its complex chemistry can help connect you to the potentials of your personal center and purpose.

**Blends well with:** Carrot seed, frankincense, ginger, helichrysum, laurel, lavandin, lavender, marjoram, neroli, palo santo, rose, rosemary ct. verbenone, spike lavender, vetiver, yarrow, ylang-ylang

**Precautions:** Can oxidize and cause skin sensitization; do not use old or oxidized oil on the skin. Also can cause sensitization when used in large amounts.

**Shelf life:** 2 to 3 years

# Eucalyptus

*Clear breathing—Expansive—Immunity*

**Common name:** Eucalyptus (pl. eucalypti), from the Greek *eucalyptos* ("well covered"), referring to the formation of its flowers

**Latin names:** *Eucalyptus globulus* (blue gum); *Eucalyptus radiata* (narrow-leaved peppermint);

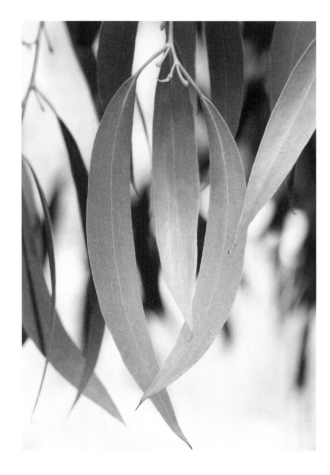

*Eucalyptus dives* (broad-leaved peppermint); *Corymbia citriadora* (lemon-scented, formally known as *Eucalyptus citriadora*)

**Botanical family:** Myrtaceae, the myrtle family, which ranges from woody shrubs to large, very tall trees. Most are tropical to subtropical plants and do well in temperate areas, often providing shade, but some species are well adapted to desert areas. *E. reg-*

*nans,* also known as the giant gum tree or mountain ash, found in Victoria and Tasmania, is the tallest known flowering plant on earth, reaching heights as great as 300 feet. There are more than 700 varieties of eucalypti, 500 of which produce essential oils (Mojay 1997). Other members of this family include tea tree and clove.

**Attributes:** Eucalyptus is all about air! Assists the respiratory system the most, but also helps you to reach above and beyond the tethers of stagnant muck within your body or emotions. (Indeed, when planted in swampy areas, eucalyptus dries the soil, transferring liquids up and out!)

**Character:** *E. globulus*, like its cousins, is quite tall, growing to 180 feet high or higher. When mature, has long, glossy pointed leaves and fragrant white flowers. As a younger plant, has rounded blue-green leaves. Australian aborigines have long used eucalyptus medicinally for wound care and as a fumigant, and it is a component in Ayurveda and Traditional Chinese Medicine (especially for lung qi). In Western medicine, often found in cough and cold medications. Steam distilled, its clear to pale yellow oil is cooling to the senses.

**Unique aroma:** Camphoraceous, minty, spicy, pungent, refreshing, resinous, woody. Other species have an additional peppermint (*E. dives*) or lemon (*E. citriadora*) scent, but always entwined with the scent of camphor.

**Aromatic note:** Top

**Part of plant used for essential oils:** Leaves and twigs

**Countries of origin:** Native to Australia, Tasmania,

## Diffuser Blend for Cold and Flu Season
### (use for adults and children age 6 or older)

Add to a water diffuser:

1 drop laurel

1 drop Roman chamomile

1 drop *Eucalyptus radiata*

Diffuse up to 30 minutes for adults. For ages 6 and up, diffuse for up to 15 minutes, turning the diffuser off for 1 to 2 hours before running again. Do not use with children under 6.

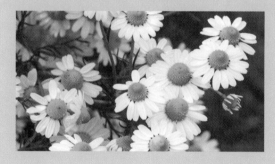

and nearby islands, now found in many parts of the world, including the United States. China is now an exporter of eucalyptus oil.

**Special chemical properties:** *E. globulus* contains 1,8 cineole (70 to 80%), α-pinene, and limonene, which support the respiratory system.

**Actions:** Antibacterial, anti-infectious, antifungal, antiviral, central nervous system suppressant (in large doses and with young children), decongestant, fever reducer, immunity tonic, insect repellent, topical circulatory stimulant (rubefacient)

**Uses** (*Extremely beneficial in a diffuser to support all the following systems*)**:**

- *Physically:* Enhances immune system function as a whole and stimulates circulation within the body. Well known for reducing and ridding phlegm and congestion from the lungs and sinuses, as well as being strongly anti-infectious. With its expectorant and decongestant qualities and a distinct camphoraceous aroma, helps trigger the limbic system to associate relief with the drying actions. Diffuse for respiratory relief while providing immunity support. *E. radiata*, which has a softer scent than (and blends well with) *E. globulus*, is useful for viral infections; *E. dives* is used for mucous colitis; *E. citriadora* is a cooling antirheumatic. Also helpful for muscular aches and pains, especially associated with coughs or muscle overuse. Use in blends designed for sprain care, and to assist in relief from shingles and chickenpox (low dilutions; use caution with children age 5 or younger).
- *Mentally:* Eucalyptus's clear fragrance stimulates the mind, aids concentration, and promotes clear thinking while supporting deep breaths.
- *Emotionally:* Clears negative emotions, opens the pathway to harmonized energy while calming the emotional nervous system, and allevi-

ates grief and sorrow, in a sense drying excess tears, while supporting the healthy letting-go of anything holding you down.

- *Spiritually:* According to the Five Element Theory in Traditional Chinese Medicine, to have clear lungs allows the spirit to create with long-term vision into the future, appropriately letting go of all that is no longer needed, opening the heart, perceiving a wider perspective on life.

**Blends well with:** Black pepper (for added warmth), cedarwood, chamomile, geranium, grapefruit, juniper berry, laurel, lavender, lemon, marjoram, melissa, rosemary, sandalwood, Scots pine

**Precautions:** As with all essential oils, eucalyptus oils can have serious effects on children. Note in particular that high concentrations of eucalyptus may suppress the central nervous system in both children and adults, causing slowed breathing, nau-

sea, and dizziness. If your pediatrician approves the use, you will still want to limit exposure by using a diffuser and allowing no more than 10 to 15 minutes at a time for children under age 5 and turning off the diffuser for 1 to 2 hours before running again. Do not apply topically in concentrations of more than 0.5% for children younger than 3 and be sure not to apply to children's faces, hands, feet, or anything else that could end up in their mouths. Consult a qualified aromatherapist to determine an appropriate dilution (which is likely to be 1% or less). Be particularly wary of preformulated blends that include eucalyptus.

Do not use eucalyptus oil if you have a seizure disorder or asthma. Avoid using in closed spaces, to prevent overdosing on the vapors. Always dilute to no more than 20% in a carrier oil to apply topically in adults. *E. dives* eucalyptus is not recommended for use with pregnant women. Note that eucalyptus is very potent and can potentially counteract homeopathic remedies.

**Shelf life:** 2 to 3 years

# Laurel
*Clean—Open—Confidence*

**Common names:** Laurel, bay laurel, Also known as sweet bay (different from California bay leaf oil, derived from *Pimenta rosemosa*, used in bay rum and sometimes called West Indian bay oil).

**Latin name:** *Laurus nobilis* ("praise" and "noble"/"renowned")

**Botanical family:** Lauraceae; includes aromatic

plants such as cinnamon, ravintsara and ravensara, litsea, and rosewood.

**Attributes:** Laurel gives people the feeling of a clear head and clear thoughts, and promotes working with others while having the space to be free in expression. Removes obstacles of stuckness, especially those connected to respiratory concerns or stagnant thoughts.

**Character:** An upright evergreen tree, sometimes cultivated as a shrub, growing anywhere from 20 to 60 feet in height, with leaves that branch out in an identifiable lanceolate shape. Adorned with small clusters of yellow flowers and then berries. Mostly tropical and subtropical, yet can grow in harsh conditions. Historically equated with love, esteem, and as a sign of success in the arts. In ancient Greece, laurel leaves were placed under pillows to stimulate prophetic dreams and were burnt as a visionary herb by priestesses at the temple of Delphi. Greeks also considered laurel an herb of protection (Mojay 1997). The Greek god Apollo considered this plant sacred and wore a crown of its leaves. Aromatherapist Gabriel Mojay shared that in medieval times, scholars and graduates of secondary education wore wreaths of laurel leaves upon their head, called *bacca laurea*, which is derived from the French term *baccalaureate*, or bachelor's degree (1997). Used in medicines from Galen (AD 165) to stimulate the liver and clear the body as a diuretic, as well as for rheumatism and edema.

**Unique aroma:** Clear, warm, cinnamon-like note, medicinal, sweet, crisp, spicy, fresh, clean, light

**Aromatic note:** Top to mid

**Part of plant used for essential oils:** Both dried and fresh leaves

**Countries of origin:** Originally from the Mediterranean, found in Morocco, France, and Croatia. Modern-day gardeners can grow laurel in a pot as a houseplant.

**Special chemical properties:** Contains 1,8 cineole, which gives that clear air scent, opening your airways.

**Actions:** Analgesic, antibacterial, antimicrobial, antiseptic, antispasmodic, antiviral, boosts immune system, calms nervous system, expectorant, fungicide

**Uses:**

- *Physically:* Assists the respiratory system; can be used in cold and flu seasons. Considered a drying oil; therefore, treats mucus conditions, including deep sinus mucus where the nose appears to be dry, and acts as an expectorant. Supportive in blends used for muscle and joint aches and pains or arthritis. Aids in circulatory stimulation to move blood peripherally and cerebrally. An immunity booster, as well as a stimulant to lymphatic movement. Can be a nervous system tonic, including providing headache relief. Used in an abdominal massage blend, can help relieve flatulence, bloating, and/or slow digestion. Can act as an astringent in skin blends designed for oily skin or acne. In Traditional Chinese Medicine, assists with circulation of qi, the vital force within.

## Air Freshener
### (room mist and linen spray)

In a 4-ounce PET plastic bottle or glass bottle with a pump, add the following essential oils to 4 ounces of 190 proof alcohol (see note):

3 drops laurel

3 drops cypress

6 drops grapefruit, mandarin, or sweet orange

*Note: Alternatively, if necessary, substitute vodka for 190 proof alcohol, and shake each time before misting. Vodka disperses just slightly less than 190 proof alcohol (hence the need to shake), which disperses completely. If using 190 proof alcohol in linen sprays, 25 to 50% alcohol to 75 to 50% distilled water is safe enough to keep bacteria from forming. Caution: Do not store or spray near an open flame.*

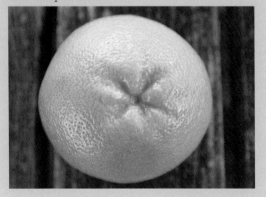

- *Mentally:* Clear thoughts are supported with increased circulation and deeper breaths. Laurel can be helpful in a blend designed for focus and concentration.
- *Emotionally:* Can help unstick emotions, especially thoughts tied to past experiences, lift you from heaviness and overwhelming emotions, and bring scattered energy to your center. Include in a blend when grief and old thoughts are present. Put a few drops in a diffuser to not only clear the air for mental support, but to dispel a heavy, stagnant feeling.
- *Spiritually:* Providing emotional support and benefits similar to those of rosemary, laurel can bring a sense of purpose and focus to the forefront. Connected to the symbolism of higher education related to a bay wreath around the head, can connect you with higher thinking and self-potential, opening the doorway to your own intuition.

**Blends well with:** Coriander, cypress, *Eucalyptus dives*, *E. radiata*, *E globulus*, frankincense, grapefruit, juniper berry, lemon, mandarin, marjoram, niaouli, palo santo, peppermint, pine, Roman chamomile, rosemary ct. cineole (for memory/concentration), rosemary ct. verbenone, and sweet orange.

**Precautions:** Do not use with children under age 5 (Shutes). Maximum concentration should be 0.5% in a total blend for general use (Tisserand and Young 2014). Laurel is very drying, so don't overdo in blends used for inhalation.

**Shelf life:** 2 to 3 years

# Patchouli

*Deep—Comforting—Connecting*

**Common name:** Patchouli

**Latin name:** *Pogostemon cablin*

**Botanical family:** Lamiaceae, often referred to as the mint family, a group of herbs and small shrubs, including lavender, melissa, mint, basil, rosemary and thyme. Most originated in the Mediterranean, but they are now found around the world, many grown in culinary and home gardens.

**Attributes:** Represents the ancient qualities of being human—survival, perseverance, depth, and the sensual and primal energies. Helps the deepest part of body, mind, and spirit come together. Patricia Davis describes patchouli well as "valuable for 'dreamers' and people who tend to neglect or feel detached from their physical bodies" (1998). Patchouli's fragrance can be an acquired aroma—literally: it is one of the very few essential oils that improves with age, deep-

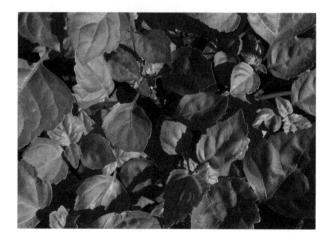

ening and mellowing. After five years or longer, its aroma is much different from that of a freshly distilled batch.

**Character:** A perennial herb growing up to 3 feet tall, with dark green aromatic leaves and small, pale pink tubular flowers. Historically, has been used in Ayurvedic, traditional Chinese, and Greek medicine as well as in Japan and Malaysia, both topically and for internal medicinal uses. Has been used for everything from snake bite to colds, halitosis, and abdominal pain. Was introduced to Victorian England in imported fabrics and shawls from India. Scenting linens with patchouli has been considered helpful in preventing pathogens and disease agents from spreading. Found modern fame as a scent as in the 1960s and early '70s in the United States. Widely used in perfumes, as a base, and for its role as a fixative for blends and synergies. The steam-distilled oil ranges in color from red-brown to pale yellow to green, depending on where the plant is grown and how it is processed. Excellent for topical use.

**Unique aroma:** Spicy, smoky, woody, sweet, rich, strong, earthy, warm, musky. Some have described patchouli as smelling like goats, musty attics, leathery, sweaty human beings, or old coats (Tisserand 1977 [1990]). Ironically, can help mask bad smells.

**Aromatic note:** Base

**Part of plant used for essential oils:** Leaves (usually slightly fermented before distillation)

**Countries of origin:** Tropical Asia and Brazil; now found around the globe

**Actions:** Antidepressant, anti-inflammatory, antimicrobial, antiviral, aphrodisiac, astringent, deodorant, digestive, relieves gas, soothes the nervous system, stimulant, tonic

**Uses:**

- *Physically:* Helps aging skin, inflamed skin, acne, athlete's foot, wrinkles, scar tissue, and cellulite. Particularly useful for stress- and hormone-related skin problems; also as an astringent. Promotes localized circulation; good for varicose veins, hemorrhoids, and edema. Include in blends designed for frigidity, menstrual cramps, low sex drive, and impotence. In addition, boosts the immune system with antibacterial, antifungal, and antiviral actions. Acts as a lymphatic and prostatic decongestant. Relieves joint and muscle pain within the musculoskeletal system. Try in your mosquito repellent blend.
- *Mentally:* Due to its centering attributes, use when confusion, poor concentration, or hyperactivity is present in the mind. Its fragrance will enhance your creativity and imagination during problem solving and study.
- *Emotionally:* When the heaviness of emotion, such as depression, permeates the heart, this oil serves as an antidepressant and also alleviates the fast vibrations of anxiety. It is historically and commonly added to aphrodisiac blends, working well with neroli, jasmine, or rose.
- *Spiritually:* Considered to be grounding, centering, meditative, and calming. Can help

## Romance Blend
### (diffuser)

Add to a water diffuser:

2 drops patchouli

2 drops neroli

1 drop jasmine (optional; this is a very expensive oil)

1 drop rose otto, or rose-scented essential oils, such as rose geranium or palmarosa (optional)

1 drop cardamom

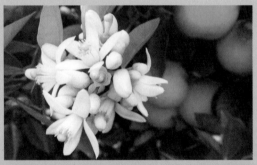

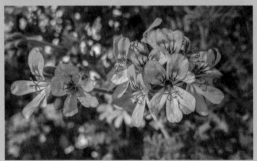

access intuitive and empathetic abilities. Jade Shutes describes patchouli nicely as being "very sensual, seducing you into accepting your body's needs" (2016), and I would add, on all levels. Try blending with palo santo, ylang-ylang, or a little bit of sweet orange or lavender.

**Blends well with:** Bergamot, black pepper, cardamom, cedarwood, chamomile, cinnamon, clary sage, clove, coriander, cypress, frankincense, geranium, ginger, grapefruit, helichrysum, jasmine, lavender, lemongrass, lime, mandarin, neroli, oakmoss, opopanax, orange, rose, sandalwood, valerian, vetiver, ylang-ylang

**Precautions:** It is important to note that this oil stimulates the nervous system in small amounts; whereas in larger doses, it acts as a sedative. Can be a sensitizer on the skin of some people; use wisely, in dilution always (5% or less).

**Shelf life:** 4 to 8+ years (patchouli gets better with age and may even have a longer life span if properly stored)

# Peppermint

*Cooling—Digestive—Awakening*

**Common Name:** Peppermint

**Latin name:** *Mentha* x *piperita L*. (The *x*, not usually spoken, is understood to mean "hybrid.")

**Botanical family:** Lamiaceae, the mint family; cousins include melissa, basil, patchouli, and spearmint.

**Attributes:** Like its roots reaching outward within the soil, and its leaves providing the fresh breath of clean air, peppermint can invigorate your mind and body. People often associate its flavor and scent with toothpaste, candy, or chewing gum.

**Character:** A natural hybrid of two aromatic mint plants—*M. spicata* (spearmint) and *M. aquatica* (water mint), peppermint is a perennial herb growing up to 3 feet tall with dark green, oval, distinctly toothed leaves and small, purple-pink flowers. Known for its roots' tendency to spread, oftentimes taking over an area of garden or natural habitat. Has been used in Eastern and Western medicines as teas, herbs, foods, and oils for digestive ailments, flatulence, nausea, headaches, and muscle cramps. Egyptians, Romans, and Greeks used this plant for scent as well as for medicinal purposes, even wearing it (or others of the *Mentha* species) as a crown and including it in decorative sprays, according to Pliny. The leaves are distilled

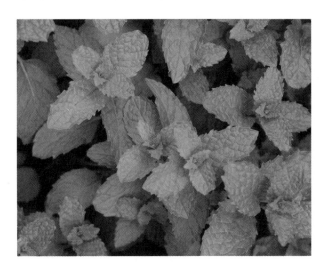

into a clear pale yellow oil. Can be both warming and cooling, sometimes confusing the initial sensation, but ultimately cooling as an essential oil.

**Unique aroma:** Fresh, menthol, clean, cool, strong, refreshing, stimulating, awakening

**Aromatic note:** Top to mid

**Part of plant used for essential oils:** Leaves

**Countries of origin:** Reportedly native to the Mediterranean, Asia, and India, yet found and distilled in many temperate climates, including France, England, and the United States (which produces more than 80% of the world's supply)

**Special chemical properties:** A complex chemical combination, best known for its menthol and menthone content that give it its distinctive flavor, aroma, and cooling action on the body.

**Actions:** Analgesic, antibacterial, anti-inflammatory, antispasmodic, antimicrobial, decongestive, digestive, expectorant, relieves coughs

**Uses:**

- *Physically:* Just as its roots travel readily through the soil, peppermint can assist the circulation of the body, both blood and lymph, where it has become slowed. Useful for varicose veins, Raynaud's disease, and lymphatic drainage (massage). Also eases digestive ailments, such as motion sickness, nausea, stomach discomfort and cramps, excess gas, irritable bowel syndrome, postsurgical nausea, and to relax a spastic colon. Aids those with chronic fatigue syndrome, spasms, aches, and pains, and fibromyalgia, and can reduce swelling and pain from sprains, strains, carpal tunnel syndrome, and sciatica. Try with clary sage, cypress, and/or lavender to alleviate menstrual discomfort. Use in a steam inhaler (1 to 2 drops max) to clear airways (keep your eyes closed as the fumes can be irritating!). Works well with eucalyptus and laurel to dry out hot, stuck phlegm and mucus from colds and flu. Commonly used to ease migraines and headaches, and as an insect repellent. Used in low doses (0.5%), can relieve itching.

- *Mentally:* Energizing and awakening to the mental facilities, opening concentration and focus, clearing thoughts and relieving the "blahs." Use alone or with lemon, lime, or orange to refresh and revive. Add to a personal inhaler blend and keep in your purse, bag, or car when traveling, to quell nausea, and as an antibacterial preventative in winter as well as a mind support.

- *Emotionally:* Add when creating uplifting synergies. Peppermint inspires deep breathing (best through your nose), which is a great trigger for the parasympathetic ("rest and rejuvenate") nervous system, relaxing nervousness and depression,

> How does peppermint differ from spearmint? Peppermint is much higher in menthol, whereas spearmint has higher carvone and minimal menthol, thus distinguishing these herbs' scent and use. Spearmint is considered milder.

> ## Good Morning Wake-Up
>
> Add to a water room diffuser:
>
> 2 drops peppermint
>
> 2 drops sweet orange or grapefruit
>
> Diffuse up to 30 minutes for adults. Do not use with children under 6. For ages 6 and up, diffuse 5 to 15 minutes if your child's pediatrician approves.

especially when you are in resistance or overwhelmed with moving forward (think of mint's roots reaching out, to help you move outward from your initial spot and to share with others).

- *Spiritually:* When the spirit feels free to express with an uplifting connection, so might it feel a freedom from pain and emotional distress. Peppermint can bring about calm awareness and stimulating awakeness, cooling the heat of excess friction.

**Blends well with:** Clary sage, *Eucalyptus radiata*, *E. globulus*, fennel, hyssop ct. cineole, juniper berry, laurel, lemon, *Litsea cubeba*, niaouli, ravintsara, rosemary ct. cineole, spearmint, thyme ct. geraniol, thyme ct. linalool, thyme ct. thymol

**Precautions:** Do not use more than 5% in a dilution (adult). Maximum dilution of 0.5% for children ages three to five. Peppermint is contraindicated in pregnancy and for use with children under three (in all forms, including diffusion). Avoid peppermint when breastfeeding as some mothers report a decrease in their milk supply when using peppermint. Be aware that preformulated or proprietary blends may include peppermint; read labels and avoid the blend if peppermint is listed in the ingredients. Peppermint must never be used near the faces or chests of children because it can suppress the central nervous system. Inhalation in large doses can result in dizziness, confusion, muscle weakness, nausea, and double vision. Can cause sensitivity to the skin, such as rashes, contact dermatitis, and eye irritation (from vapors). Use with caution, use common sense, and use proper dilution—less is more!

*Do not ingest!* Ingestion can be fatal.

Those with sensitivity to this herb may want to proceed with caution with both peppermint and *E. dives* (a.k.a. broad-leaved eucalyptus peppermint) oils. Avoid undiluted application especially to open wounds and sensitive skin.

**Shelf life:** 2 to 4 years

# Pine

*Breathe—Clear—Clean*

**Common names:** Pine has many species within its genus, including Scots pine (a.k.a. Scotch pine) and piñon pine (a.k.a. pinyon pine).

**Latin names:** Scots pine: *Pinus sylvestris*; piñon pine: *Pinus edulis*

**Botanical family:** Pinaceae, known for the great trees, such as pines, spruces, firs, cedars, hemlocks, and larches. Other than the ocean itself being the largest biome (major life zone), this family contributes to the largest land biome on the planet, the boreal forest. The boreal forest covers the Northern Hemisphere from North America to Eurasia, but this family can be found in places around the planet, ranging from the native forests of the deserts to swamps to high mountain regions. Trees in this family can range from 6 to 328 feet tall, and most are evergreens. Cousins include ponderosa pine, Corsican pine, and maritime pine, which are also made into essential oils.

**Attributes:** One of the most beloved scents from antiquity, pine helps the planet breathe freely, being both clean smelling and versatile in lung and environmental air qualities.

**Character:** Its needle-shape leaves, unique and different from those of other trees, remind you that

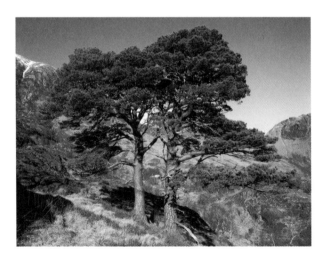

small things can have a big impact. Indigenous to the warmer deserts of the southwest United States, Piñon Pine has a history of Native American use for food (pine nuts), medicines, fire, and materials. Native Americans honor symbiotic relationships just as piñon pine relies on birds to help propagate its seeds in the desert. As an essential oil, Piñon Pine is milder and sweeter than some of its crisp, piney cousins. Scots pine is the most widely dispersed pine in the boreal forest in northern Europe and used for tar, turpentine, timber, and essential oils. Greeks and Egyptians sought Scots pine for ceremony and medicine, to stave off pests, and to fill mattresses and pillows. It is also generally considered the most useful and safest therapeutically of all the pines (Shutes 2016).

**Unique aroma:** Fresh, clean, forestlike, coniferous, high secret sweet note in some species, turpenic, balsam, soft-fruity, resinous, earthy, and piney

**Aromatic note:** Top to mid

**Part of plant used for essential oils:** Needles primarily; in some species, the odorous resin is also used, along with the cone; in lower-quality distillations, the wood is used.

**Countries of origin:** Found in the Northern Hemisphere across the world, in Eurasia, and branching outward, but the oils are primarily distributed from France (Scots pine) and the United States (piñon pine); thrives in the deserts of Arizona, Colorado, New Mexico, and Utah.

**Special chemical properties:** Its high levels of α-

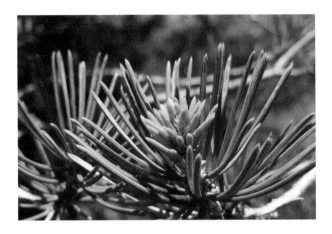

pinene gives pine its distinctive aroma and its therapeutic benefits.

**Actions:** Analgesic, antibacterial, antibiotic, anti-infectious, anti-inflammatory, antifungal, antimicrobial, assists in opening lungs and air pathways, expectorant, soothes nerves

**Uses:**

- *Physically:* Can help you breathe easily and openly, clearing away mucus. Use for all respiratory concerns—coughs, sore throats, allergies, bronchitis, or catarrh, as well as to improve atmospheric air qualities. Can soothe nervous tension by encouraging deeper breaths and therefore greater intake of oxygen into the body. Due to its turpenic action, good for muscle and joint pain, including arthritis, rheumatism, and stiffness (try with a little black pepper, peppermint, rosemary, marjoram, and/or lavender). If there are circulatory needs, will increase stimulation and movement. Can also help with excess fluid in tissues, such as edema.

- *Mentally:* Clarity of thought is important; by helping you breathe well, pine can encourage more oxygen, thus delivering parasympathetic rest and rejuvenation with lightness and ease. Can ease mental fatigue, heavy thoughts, and stressful whirling in the mind. Smelling this clean, clear fragrance is recommended in times of too much "city life," to reconnect with your inner nature without the mental clutter.

- *Emotionally:* When you are overwhelmed with anxiety, depression, or melancholy, think of pine's tall trunks rising above all the dust, its potent, powerful leaves piercing past the heaviness of damp emotions, opening the way to feeling refreshed and relaxed, and cleansing away any nonbeneficial thoughts and emotions. For emotional uses, works nicely with palo santo and lavender, as well as the uplifting nature of citrus to inner calm.

- *Spiritually:* Helps you distinguish between your purpose and taking on tasks meant for others. Pine helps you let go, set healthy boundaries, and find your freedom. Adding to a blend designed for meditation can help open up the breath and mind.

**Blends well with:** Balsam fir, bergamot, black spruce, cedarwood, clary sage, corkbark fir, Corsican pine, cypress, Douglas fir, lemon, euca-

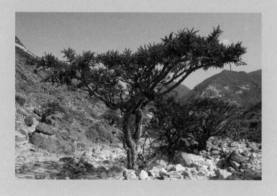
lyptus, frankincense, grapefruit, lavender, mandarin, niaouli, peppermint, petigrain, piñon pine, ponderosa pine, ravensara, ravintsara, Rocky Mountain pine, rosalina, rosemary ct. cineole, sandalwood, Scots pine, sweet orange, tea tree, white fir, ylang-ylang

**Precautions:** Use in a maximum 1 to 3% dilution

when applied to the skin, as can be irritating to the skin if too high. Do not use old or oxidized oils, which can irritate and dry out the skin. Be mindful when using with those who experience asthma, as the same constituents that help to move mucus may be too strong for asthmatic lungs.

**Shelf life:** 1 to 3 years

## Silver Fir

*Purifier—Creative—Open*

**Common name:** Silver fir

**Latin name:** *Abies alba*

**Botanical family:** Pinaceae family, which includes pines, spruces, firs, cedars, hemlocks, and larches. As is the *Pinus* genus of resinous trees, fir is a source of turpentine. This entire botanical family is very connected to planetary support and protectors of the air in the earth's atmosphere, especially in the Northern Hemisphere.

**Attributes:** Forest trees have a deep knowing about the environment around themselves and their place in it, and thus can help you connect to this intuitiveness about yourself and your purpose. One of the respiratory helpers, assists in setting boundaries and seals emotional and mental wounds just as does its resin.

**Character:** Usually grows from 98 to a little less than 200 feet in height. The bark is filled with resinous canals. This resin is tapped from mature trees at least 60 to 80 years old; like that of its pine cousins, it is highly valued for its turpentine

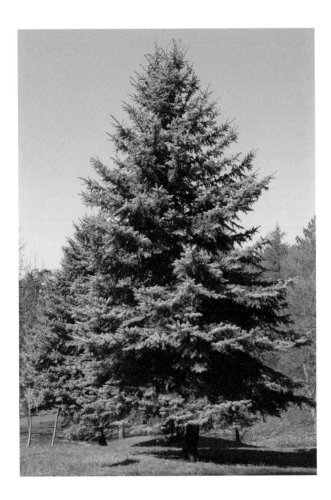

and oleo-resin residue, often called rosin oil. (If you have ever played a stringed instrument, you may be familiar with the rosin for your bow that comes from this family of Pinaceae trees.) The resins are often used to create varnishes, lacquers, and solvents, and for caulking ships. Historically,

the oil has been added to perfumes and medicines; in Europe, has been used for fever, muscular, and rheumatic pain.

**Unique aroma:** Fresh, delicate, fruity, balsamic, heady, green incense, resinous, turpenic

**Aromatic note:** Top to mid

**Part of plant used for essential oils:** Needles

**Countries of origin:** Distilled oils come from France, Albania, and Canada, but firs can be found in Europe, North and Central America, northern Africa, and Asia.

**Special chemical properties:** Its high levels of d-limonene (up to 34%) and $\alpha$-pinene (up to 37%), and camphene and $\beta$-pinene support its therapeutic actions.

**Actions:** Analgesic, antibacterial, antimicrobial, antiseptic, antiviral, decongestant, expectorant, immunity booster, stimulant

**Uses:**

- *Physically:* Clears airways in times of bronchitis, respiratory infections, allergies, congested breathing, sinus issues, and colds and flu, especially when excess mucus or phlegm is involved. Add to your diffusers and personal inhalers to assist in room or travel lung support. You may include this oil in your blends to quell asthma. Due to its analgesic properties, can relieve sore muscles and joint aches.
- *Mentally:* Clean air naturally promotes a deep breath. When you bring in purified air, the mind benefits with clarity and calmness in focus.

145

## Clean Air

Add to a water room diffuser:

2 to 3 drops silver fir

2 to 3 drops *Eucalyptus radiata*

- *Emotionally:* The natural affinity the forest has on calming the mind and emotional heart is in part due to its fresh scent. The components in silver fir's chemical makeup, along with that of other amazing forest trees, contain natural relaxers and feel-good constituents encouraging deep breaths, letting the hustle and bustle of life recede while enjoying the present moment. This essential oil has uplifting and soothing properties.
- *Spiritually:* All the forest trees in this family encourage awareness of the environment. Trees are considered wisdom keepers. Add this essential oil to synergies intended for intuitive and meditative moments. Be open to deeper perspectives when connecting with this essential oil.

**Blends well with:** Bergamot, cedarwood, chamomiles, cypress, eucalyptus, firs, frankincense, helichrysum, juniper berry, laurel, lavender, lemon, neroli, palo santo, patchouli, pine, rosalina, rosemary, spruce

**Precautions:** Do not use oxidized oils. Risk of skin sensitization is increased with oxidized oils. Store in the refrigerator. You can add a drop of vitamin E to a silver fir blend if it is to be used topically.

**Shelf life:** 1 to 3 years

## Rosemary

*Invigorating—Tonic—Awakening*

**Common names:** Rosemary; chemotypes include rosemary ct. cineole and rosemary ct. verbenone (Two additional chemotypes not covered in this book are ct. camphor and ct. borneol.)

**Latin name:** *Rosmarinus officinalis* ("dew of the sea," due to its affinity with water)

**Botanical family:** Lamiaceae, which includes lavender, mint, sage, thyme, melissa, and patchouli. Rosemary is found all over the world, in different altitudes and terrains, including many backyard and culinary gardens.

**Attributes:** Inviting to the senses, has the ability to soothe the body and sharpen the mind at the same time. Enhances memory, produces clear air, promotes a "you-can-do-it" attitude.

**Character:** A well-known shrub used for culinary, medicinal, and tonic preparations, grows anywhere from 3 to 8 feet in height (some species, such as creeping rosemary, have ability to branch out). Gentle light blue flowers decorate its flat, needle-like, odorous leaves, which are thick with easily available resinous aromatic oils. Has been used in sickrooms and hospitals to clean and purify the air, as well as for general calming of the overwhelmed mind, inducing brain function through its scent and soothing sore muscles topically. Has historical asso-

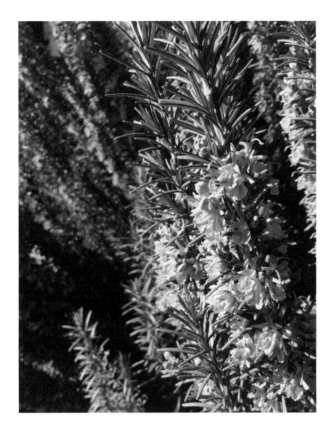

**Aromatic note:** Top to mid

**Part of plant used for essential oils:** Sprigs and flowering tops consisting of the leaves, flowers, and stems

**Countries of origin:** Originally from the Mediterranean regions and coastal areas, now cultivated throughout Europe, various areas in Africa, the Middle East, and the United States.

**Special chemical properties:** Rosemary's chemical composition varies depending on its growing conditions, the soil, the sun, the moon, the rain, and the air, creating unique chemotypes (see pages 57–58). Rosemary ct. verbenone has high verbenone and camphor levels, and $\alpha$-pinene. Rosemary ct. 1,8 cineole has marked levels of 1,8 cineole, which support memory and cognitive function, and also gives it a sharper aroma than verbenone.

**Actions:** Analgesic, anti-inflammatory, anti-infectious, antiseptic, antispasmodic, breaks up mucous, cognitive stimulant, decongestant, expectorant, muscle relaxant (cineole), stimulant, tonic, wound healing (verbenone)

**Uses:**

- *Physically:* Add to muscle and joint analgesics or soothing massage topical tonics (along with lavender, black pepper, and marjoram). A little bit in a massage can relieve muscle stiffness and general body malaise. Can boost immunity by clearing the air, purifying it from pathogens, and relieving congestion, bronchitis, and coughs (especially when used with eucalyptus, peppermint, and cedarwood). Aids in circulatory sup-

ciations with good luck, loyalty, friendship, and love; its being a protection herb intertwines folklore and reality, as clear thinking and strong body will help with good decisions. Has been admired by European cultures, Greeks, and Romans for health of body and mind, in Egypt in the form of incense, and as inspiration for poetry and art.

**Unique aroma:** Sharp, strong, fresh, camphoraceous, vibrant, awakening, brisk, penetrating, balsamic, woody, medicinal

# Scalp Tonic

In a small container, combine 1 ounce (2 tablespoons) of gently warmed coconut oil, or jojoba if scalp is dry, (do not microwave) and:

6 to 7 drops rosemary ct. verbenone

1 drop rosemary ct. cineole

1 drop frankincense (Boswellia carteri)

1 drop juniper berry

1 drop rosalina

Add a small amount of this blend to small sections of the scalp in small, circular, mindful motions, moving the hair out of the way as you move on to each new location. Massage the scalp first, then apply any remaining residue on your hands to the hair strands. Leave on for 30 minutes to overnight (cover your head with a plastic hair cap). Do not drench your head in water to wash; instead, wash by first applying shampoo to the "dry" (oiled) hair, adding water only by using your hands. Once a lather is built, then apply a steady stream of water to rinse the hair. Repeat as needed.

port by creating warm, stimulating movement locally and mentally. Try in carrier oil scalp rubs to stimulate circulation of the scalp, as a hair tonic, to give a head massage, and to stimulate the mind as well. Can be used for skin-related issues, such as dandruff, hair loss, rashes, eczema, and dermatitis. Use in a carrier oil for abdominal massages to ease gas and bloating and to promote healthy digestion.

- *Mentally:* Assists with cognitive and memory function; helps older persons by promoting clear, open thoughts and recalling information; and relieves mental exhaustion. Can provide focus in times when mental concentration and recall are important, such as during study or organizing. Rosemary ct. cineole is especially useful for memory and cognitive support. Personal and room diffusers are phenomenal for this purpose.
- *Emotionally:* Clear thoughts and clear air help soothe the nervous systems of fatigue, open the chest, and open the heart to positive thoughts and feelings. When you think clearly, you can feel clearly, boosting confidence, assisting with coping mechanisms in stressful situations. Rosemary can help individuals who tend to live in a whirl of emotions and thoughts, lacking the self-esteem to set boundaries and pursue personal purpose. Try rosemary ct. verbenone for emotional and spiritual blends.
- *Spiritually:* Just as rosemary sprigs can scent the air with just a brush against their surface, so too, can this essential oil help lift the mind and spirit upward.

**Blends well with:** Cedarwood, cypress, Eucalyptus species, fennel, grapefruit, juniper berry, laurel, lemon, lemongrass, monarda (wild bergamot), niaouli, peppermint, pine, ravensara, ravintsara, rosalina, tea tree

**Precautions:** Do not use during pregnancy, breast-feeding, or with children under 2 years of age; any history of epilepsy or seizures; or if a fever is present (can be applied after fever has gone, for antibacterial and anti-infectious properties). Keep dilution at 2% or lower.

**Shelf life:** 2 to 4 years

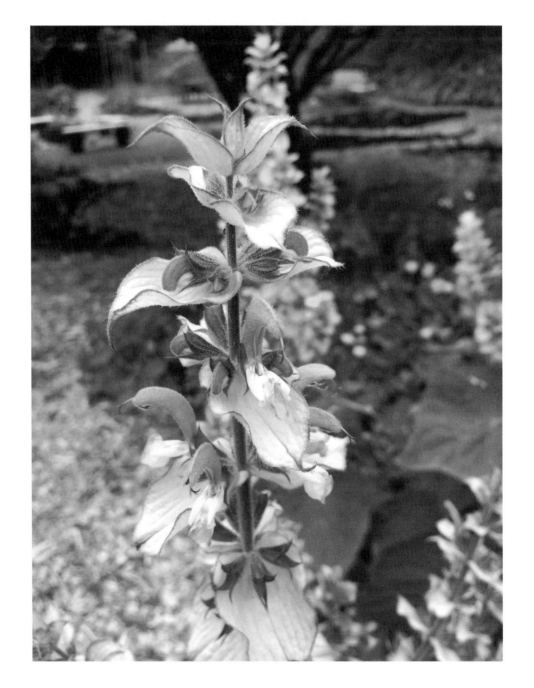

# CHAPTER 10

# Petals and Flowers

*Every flower is a soul blossoming in nature.* —Gerard de Nerval

## Calming—Soothing—Self-care

Petals and flowers denote love, creativity, free to be oneself, sensory, expressive, spontaneity, and living in the moment.

Flowers are easily the most identifiable aromatic part of a plant. Their colorful petals invite insects, animals, and birds to come closer. (Scent was the most ancient identifier of a plant—even before color!) Floral aromas range from strong and sweet, to light and soft, to spicy and robust. The physiological, psychological, emotional, and spiritual shifts and changes they induce can be beneficial to our well-being. Floral scents are historically linked with feminine, soft, nurturing, alluring, and aphrodisiac qualities, but masculine natures also benefit from their allure. In practical applications, floral essential oils can ease anxiety or an emotional heart, calm a restless mind, soothe menstrual issues, and comfort hormonal upsets.

## Clary Sage
*Euphoric—Feminine—Inviting*

**Common name:** Clary sage

**Latin name:** *Salvia sclarea*

**Botanical family:** Lamiaceae, sometimes called Labiatae; cousins include lavender, mint, rosemary, patchouli, basil, and thyme.

**Attributes:** Has a deep connection to the qualities of the female human experience and the feminine softness needed to secure her internal strength. Considered a woman's essential oil (but is beneficial to men, too). Cools frustrations, anger, and changeable moods; a balancer.

**Character:** This plant's petals come to a sharp point—perhaps why its name derives from the Greek *skleria*. *Salvia*, Latin for "to save, to heal," reflects its history of medicinal uses for both body and mind with harmonization properties. Growing 3 to 6 feet in height, depending on the species,

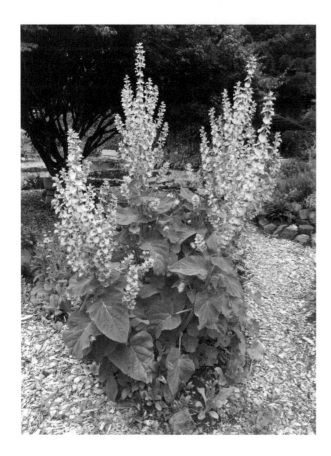

with wide leaves that are fuzzy and welcoming but nondescript compared to its flowers, which are white or soft pastels of pink, lavender, or blue thinly outlined in purple, as if barely dipped in ink. As far back as the Middle Ages, has been used for medicinal properties as an aromatic plant. Used safely, clary sage can be a wonderful oil for your needs.

**Unique aroma:** Rich, musky, reminiscent of the scent of tea, nutty, softly floral, tobacco, earthy, tannic or winelike, bittersweet, warm, with a whisper of spice

**Aromatic note:** Mid to base

**Part of plant used for essential oils:** Flowers

**Countries of origin:** Europe (France, Germany, Russia, and Italy)

**Special chemical properties:** The main chemicals are linalool (up to 20%) and linalyl acetate (up to 75%), both powerfully effective in soothing the nervous system. Chemically similar to lavender, which is considered a stronger relaxant; clary sage is more euphoric.

**Actions:** Antidepressant, antifungal, anti-inflammatory, antispasmodic, aphrodisiac, calms nervous system, relaxes the uterus and stimulates blood flow (helps with menstrual flow and during labor)

**Uses:**

- *Physically:* Aids scanty or irregular menstrual cycles, PMS, menopause, and childbirth. (Only use clary sage during childbirth if your obstetrician agrees and if you are being attended by a trained aromatherapist.) Can relieve joint aches and pains and helpful for muscle spasms, cramps, sciatica, and plantar fasciitis as well as arthritis. Regulates sebum, reducing both excess (oily) and deficient (dry) secretions on the scalp and skin, including acne, boils, ulcers, and wrinkles (often produced by dry skin); provides gentle support for mature skin. Add to blends to calm sore throats and coughs. While not

# Personal Inhaler for Stress Relief

Drop the following onto a personal inhaler cotton wick (preferably organic cotton).

3 drops clary sage

4 to 5 drops lavender

6 to 7 drops sweet orange or mandarin

For a room water diffuser:

1 drop clary sage

2 drops lavender

3 drops sweet orange or mandarin

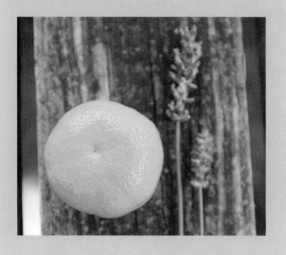

estrogenic, has been shown to have hormone-balancing effects with women.

- *Mentally:* When pain is present due to high anxiety, can calm the mind (mental), lessening the sensation of pain (body). Useful for overwork-caused exhaustion, insomnia, frigidity, hyperactivity, and mental fatigue.
- *Emotionally:* When anxiety, anger, frustration, and irritation, illusionary feelings of worry, or despondency is present, can calm the emotional storm and provide a gentle uplift of euphoria, reducing sensations of stress and soothing the indecisive, distracted heart space. Works especially well with women.
- *Spiritually:* Will connect you to your dream states, as well as induce beneficial emotional and mental contentment. Also common in aphrodisiac blends. As a harmonizer and central nervous system relaxer, connects the body, mind, emotions, and spirit into a balanced state.

**Blends well with:** Bergamot, grapefruit, jasmine, lavender, mandarin, rose, and rose-scented (palmarosa and geranium), sweet orange, ylang-ylang. To ease muscles, try with black pepper, fennel, geranium, juniper berry, lavender, lemongrass, or Roman chamomile. For deeper meditative states, combine with frankincense, palo santo, and sandalwood.

**Precautions:** Do not use clary sage if you are pregnant: it might cause premature labor. Do not drink alcohol while you are using clary sage. That combination may cause exaggeratedly intoxicated behavior and a hangover. Use a maximum dilution of

2.5% to avoid adverse skin reactions (Tisserand and Young 2014).

**Shelf life:** 4 to 5 years

# Chamomile

*Calming—Accepting—Soothing*

**Common names:** Chamomile: German chamomile, a.k.a. wild or blue chamomile; Roman chamomile, a.k.a. English chamomile

**Latin names:** German chamomile is properly listed as *Matricaria chamomilla*. Roman chamomile *Anthemis nobilis*.

**Botanical family:** Asteraceae, also known as Compositae; however, note that German and English chamomile are cousins, not siblings. You can tell by their genera: *Matricaria* is not the same as *Anthemis*. Other relatives include arnica, calendula, and helichrysum.

**Attributes:** Chamomile is calming, like napping on a hammock on a breezy, sunny day. It is also a helper, ready to steady your being, and a gentle protector.

**Character:** Both German and Roman chamomile have delicate light green leaves and white petal blooms dotted with bright yellow raised centers, resembling little daisies, another cousin (as are sunflowers). Roman chamomile flowers *and* leaves are strongly aromatic, with solid, sometimes double flower heads and feathery leaves; also, Roman has a very tiny, telltale scale between each two florets, a typical sign of a true chamomile, and a "vital characteristic of the genus *Anthemis*,"

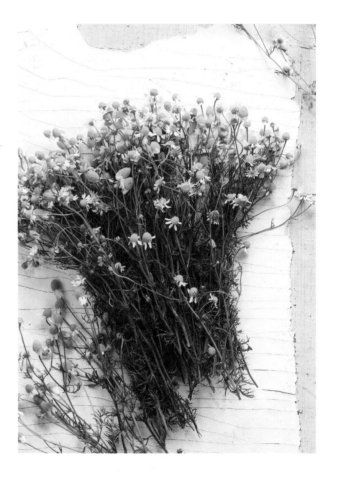

according to Mrs. Grieves. As for German chamomile, only its hollow flower heads are aromatic, its leaves are not, and instead of being between florets, overlapping scales surround the base of the flower head. Chamomile has been used for herbal infusions, tinctures, and medicinally for more than 2,500 years by Egyptian to Roman to Greek cultures to soothe skin, as a digestive, to calm the mind, and primarily as an anti-inflammatory agent.

**Unique aroma:** Roman chamomile: applelike, sweet, fruity, strong, aromatically strong, but softer than German. German chamomile: hay- or herblike, sweet, strong, tealike, grassy, aromatically strong, but more bitter or sharper than Roman.

**Aromatic note:** Roman: mid to top; German: mid to base

**Part of plant used for essential oils:** Flowers

**Countries of origin:** Roman: Europe (Italy, France, Germany, Hungary), United States, and Chile; German: Europe, North America, and Australia

**Special chemical properties:** Roman chamomile also contains ketones and esters (up to 80%), accounting for its sedative and anti-spasmodic actions. German chamomile is higher in alcohols, oxides, and trace aldehydes, and is blue due to constituents of chamazulene, hence you can remember it as the blue chamomile. German chamomile is anti-inflammatory and anti-infectious.

**Actions:** Analgesic, antimicrobial (both varieties, but especially German), cools and soothes central nervous system, antidepressant, anti-inflammatory (German), antispasmodic (Roman), digestive stimulant, sedative (Roman), reduces anxiety, relieves gas (German), wound healing

**Uses:**

- *Physically:* Both chamomile species provide support for the nervous system, inflammation, insomnia, menstrual issues, headaches, and skin concerns, such as acne. German chamomile is useful when the skin issues are a bit more heightened, such as with eczema, psoriasis, and burns, including sunburns (great mixed with aloe vera). For inflammation, both do quite nicely; however, German chamomile's chamazulene is helpful here. Use either species in a low-dilution abdominal belly rub for adults and children over the age of 5 (Butje 2017). Jade Shutes mentions German chamomile as good for more intense skin, reproductive, and anti-inflammatory situations. Roman chamomile aids with general skin and digestive concerns (2016) as well as sedative actions.

- *Mentally:* Any time an essential oil can calm the mental aspects of a person, there is great benefit. Roman chamomile can assist with calming and soothing the thoughts, in part by reducing inflammation and anxiety, which results in better coping overall.

- *Emotionally:* Calm minds and smoothed-out emotions produce better sleep. Overstimulation can be quelled with use of either chamomile (great for overactive or overstimulated kids). Inhalation can produce calming effects in diffusers, but due to the expense of these precious oils, personal inhalers as well as localized applications may prove more cost effective. (Alternatively, inhaling the fragrance of a brewed infusion [tea] of chamomile flowers can be beneficial.)

- *Spiritually:* The energy of the sunshine flows through chamomile flowers, awakening the

## Rest Well Diffuser Blend
### (safe for children over age 5 and adults)

Add the following essential oils to a water diffuser. Run the diffuser 30 minutes (10 to 15 minutes for children) before bedtime in the room you will be sleeping in:

1 to 2 drops Roman chamomile

2 drops lavender

Turn off the diffuser before you turn out the light and go to bed.

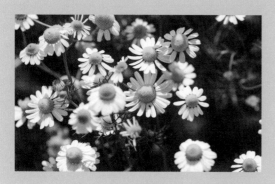

senses while calming excess energy: perfect for meditation, prayer, contemplation, and consciousness exploration. Euphoria and serenity can be accessed when the mind is quiet and the spirit is open.

**Blends well with:** Bergamot, chamomile, clary sage, cypress, elemi, frankincense, juniper berry, lavender, lemon, mandarin, melissa, neroli, patchouli, rose geranium, sweet marjoram, sweet orange, ylang-ylang

**Precautions:** The University of Maryland suggests on its Integrative Care website to avoid chamomile while pregnant, due to risk of miscarriage. If you are allergic to ragweed, daisies, asters, or chrysanthemums, or sensitive to chamomile, you probably want to avoid this oil or use extreme caution (you might be sensitive to chamomile tea, too!). Due to its sedative effects, chamomile should not be used in conjunction with other sedating substances. It may increase bleeding if used in conjunction with blood thinners. This oil is prone to oxidation; store away from light, air, and heat, preferably in a cold location, such as a refrigerator. May cause skin irritations if oxidized or if the individual is sensitive to the flower family.

Strong enough to be effective and gentle enough to use with children. Roman chamomile is an effective substitute for other antimicrobial oils, such as tea tree when using a blend with children. It can also be substituted for or used in addition to lavender. German chamomile is good for children age 5 and up. Hydrosols are excellent substitutes for essential oils for young ones under age 5.

**Shelf life:** 4 to 5 years

# Helichrysum

*Wholeness—Soothe—Repair*

**Common names:** Helichrysum (*hel-ih-KRY-sum*), from the Greek *heli* ("sun") and *chrysum* ("gold"), reflecting a value and power always "worth its weight in gold." Also known as Everlasting and Immortelle, as the blooms retain their color after being dried.

**Latin name:** *Helichrysum italicum*

**Botanical family:** Asteraceae, one of the largest flowering families in botanical nomenclature, with more than 1,100 genera and 25,000 species. Cousins include chamomile, daisies, and sunflowers as well as arnica and calendula.

**Attributes:** A significant promoter of skin health, especially after external or internal trauma to the skin; can also help you knit together a healthy foundation after emotional scars and experiences.

**Character:** Has long been used in homeopathy, as a medicinal plant, and for decoration (the dried flowers can last for years). Uses as an oil were referred to in the late 1800s and early 1900s in medicinal pharmacopoeia dispensary literature. However, helichrysum was not listed as an essential oil before the 1980s, according to Kurt Schnaubelt to the general public for use (2011). Although sometimes called "curry plant" in garden stores due to the plant's leaves' aroma, it is not the source of any curry spices.

**Unique aroma:** Warm, spicy, herbaceous, bittersweet, honeylike, currylike (especially in botanical plant form)

**Aromatic note:** Mid

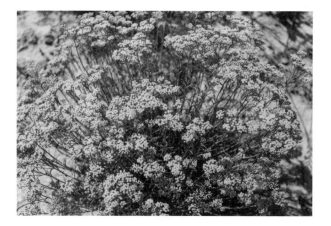

**Part of plant used for essential oils:** Flowering tops and flowers

**Countries of origin:** Originally native to the Mediterranean, now found in Italy, Corsica, Dalmatia, France, Spain, and Bosnia. (Other *Helichrysum* species grow in different parts of the world; look for *H. italicum*.)

**Special chemical properties:** Its highest component is an ester, neryl acetate (25 to 50%), which accounts for its slightly fruity-floral-honey fragrance.

**Actions:** Analgesic, anticoagulant (thus helps with bruises), antidepressant, antifungal, antispasmodic, calmative, and wound healing

**Uses:**

- *Physically:* Long used to dispel pooled blood and to aid bruised tissue and hematomas by encouraging blood flow. Comparable to the homeopathic remedy arnica, known for aiding soft tissue trauma. Considered the number one skin remedy

# Bruise Helper Gel

Add the following to 1 ounce of aloe vera gel:

4 drops helichrysum
5 drops lavender
2 drops cypress
2 drops lemon

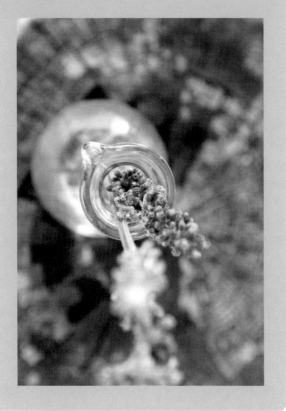

in essential oils, helpful for wound healing, cellular regeneration, dermal inflammation, aging skin, eczema and psoriasis, scar tissue, burns, and rosacea. Soothes bumps, bruises, sprains, muscle aches, or stiff arthritis. Benefits varicose veins, broken capillaries, and circulation issues (e.g., Reynaud's disease). Add to blends to relieve sinus infections, chest ailments, including bronchitis or congestion (works great combined or in rotation with rosemary ct. cineole).

- *Mentally:* Helps release overcontrolling tension of the mind and body. Irritability associated with stuck feelings can give way to freer flow within the thought process.
- *Emotionally:* Calm is this oil's middle name. Similar to chamomile in its ability to soothe emotional upsets, such as frustration, irritability, resentment, or stubbornness; however, will also help you overcome the holds of old trauma, stuck places of emotional scars or exhaustion. Gently brings in freshness, like opening a window to air out a stagnant room. Can assist with peace of mind and emotional harmony. Useful for children who are unable to find their center (hyperactivity). Use in times of much needed stress reduction and to reduce anxiety.
- *Spiritually:* The gift of clarity of mind and body and harmonized emotions promotes inner compassion and the release of old experiences. The letting-go of despair or anger opens you to the possibility of a calm center, forgiving others, and a beneficial spiritual experience.

**Blends well with:** German or Roman chamomile, rosemary ct. verbenone, rosemary ct. cineole, sweet orange, lemon, grapefruit, lavender, cistus, lavendin, rose geranium, frankincense, sandalwood, palo santo, clary sage, sweet marjoram, peppermint, patchouli, vetiver

**Precautions:** Maximum dermal use is suggested to be 0.5% (3 to 4 drops per ounce of carrier) to avoid skin irritation in sensitive individuals (Tisserand and Young 2014). Those with allergies to plants in the Asteraceae family may want to proceed with caution to avoid an unforeseen trigger.

**Shelf life:** 4 to 5 years

# Geranium, Rose

*Feminine—Relief—Love*

**Common name:** Rose geranium

**Latin names:** *Pelargonium* x *asperum* and *Pelargonium graveolens*, var. *roseum*; often listed as *Pelargonium graveolens*.

**Botanical family:** Geraniacaea, home to many herbs and shrubs. Rose geranium is but one of 280 species of the *Pelargonium* genus (*Encyclopaedia Britannica* 2000), including scented geranium sisters such as lemon, lime, and citrosa. Do not confuse with "true geraniums," from the *Geranium* genus (also in the Geraniacaea family), which disperse seeds by flinging them and grow in cooler climates. *Pelargonium* prefers temperate to warm conditions and has feathered seed pods that allow the breeze to disperse them.

**Attributes:** Soft yet powerful; cools heat from the

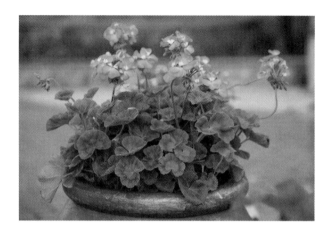

body and mind. Good to use when you cannot access rose essential oil.

**Character:** As an essential oil, possesses many of the qualities its other rose-fragrant friends do as a soother of emotions. Has a slight underlying green note within its odor, signifying its geranium nature as opposed to the rose family.

**Unique aroma:** Floral, sweet, spicy, green, herbaceous, roselike, fresh, strong, feminine, slightly citrusy

**Aromatic note:** Mid

**Part of plant used for essential oils:** Flowers and leaves (the whole plant is aromatic!)

**Countries of origin:** Native to South Africa, but found all along temperate regions of the globe. The Réunion Islands, Egypt, Madagascar, India, Morocco, and China are additional areas of essential oil production. The oils may have slight differences in scent depending on their environment.

**Actions:** Analgesic, antibacterial, anti-inflammatory,

antimicrobial, astringent, "hormone balancer" (along with clary sage), reduces anxiety, sedative, stimulating

**Uses:**

- *Physically:* Has an affinity with blends that soothe scars, acne, eczema, aging skin, rashes, and other skin irritations and inflammation. For swelling, such as sprains or bumps and bruises, combine with lavender or helichrysum. For skin issues of dryness or too much oil, can harmonize sebum production. Add to your scalp oil for hair and skin support while giving an amazing scent to your hair (best used earlier in the day rather than at night, if you find it energizes rather than relaxes you). Menstrual concerns with mood and sore muscles and joints also benefit from its use due to its cooling and anti-inflammatory action. Supports healthy lymph drainage and can be added to blends designed for circulatory and lymphatic harmony. Bring on your travels to assist with jet lag.
- *Mentally:* This oil's scent and chemical makeup are perfect for addressing anxiety, which can create a cluttered mind.
- *Emotionally:* Soothes stressful emotions; especially helpful for hormone-induced mood swings and exhaustion due to overwork. To cool hot emotions and hot feelings in your body, add to a cooling, harmonizing blend. Think of rose geranium when you need the feeling of love and support.
- *Spiritually:* Like the soft pulse of breath

## Good Night Open Heart Emotion Soother

Add to a 1-ounce container of your favorite carrier oil:

1 drop rose geranium

1 drop ylang-ylang

1 drop clary sage

2 drops bergamot, sweet orange, or neroli

2 drops lavender

Use at night before bed. If you prefer, add to an unscented lotion or cream and apply as a nighttime foot and hand cream. Gently run your fingers through your hair so any remaining residue can lightly fragrance your hair while you rest.

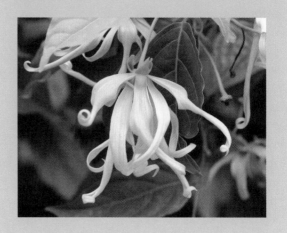

exchange, can assist in finding the harmony of life of giving and receiving. The gentleness of rose and the subtle uplifting spice of life are wrapped in its scent. Breathe with it.

**Blends well with:** Bergamot, frankincensum, jasmine, lavender, lime, mandarin, neroli, palo santo, rose, rosemary ct. verbenone, sandalwood, sweet orange

**Precautions:** Make sure to use in proper dilution, blended well, as skin irritations can result from contact of the undiluted essential oil with sensitive skin. As noted earlier, rose geranium is generally sedative, but for some it can be rejuvenating, so find out how it works best for you. Tisserand and Young suggest maximum dermal use at 17.5% (but due to fragrance intensity, you'll likely use much less).

**Shelf life:** 3 to 5 years

## Jasmine
*Softening—Seducing—Enamoring*

**Common names:** Jasmine; "moonlight of the grove" (Hindu); "queen of the night" (India)

**Latin names:** *Jasminum samba* (night-blooming); *Jasminum grandiflorum* (dawn-blooming)

**Botanical family:** Oleaceae, a family of climbers, shrubs, trees, and vines. *Jasminum* falls into its woody climber category. One familiar cousin is olive (often used as a base for herbal infused oils).

**Attributes:** Warms the senses, seduces the mind and the body, and aligns the emotions.

**Character:** A vinelike, flowering plant with star-

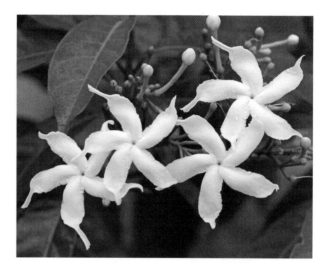

shaped, delicate white flowers. Despite the blossoms' small size, the fragrance that is released when they open is strong and sweet without holding back. Most fragrant during August and September. As far back as the empires of Asia, has been used to scent perfumes and medicines alike. It takes more than 3.5 million of these gently hand-picked flowers to create just 1 pound. Therefore, second to rose, this is one of the most expensive natural fragrances to produce. Do not use synthetic copies of this scent as they do not offer the same bioactive components for positive experiences and benefits.

**Unique aroma:** Night-blooming jasmine has a rather rich, exotic, heavily sweet smell, with sultry and fruity notes. Dawn-blooming jasmine has a sweet, floral, fruity smell, but with softer and lighter notes than its moon-illuminated cousin.

**Aromatic note:** Base

# Jasmine Smiles Personal Perfume

Create a synergy first in a 10 ml roller bottle with its roller ball removed:

1 drop jasmine

1 drop clary sage

2 drops rose geranium

2 drops lavender

2 drops mandarin

1 drop patchouli

2 drops champa herbal infused carrier oil (optional)

6 drops jasmine herbal infused carrier oil (optional)

Jojoba carrier oil

Allow the oils to meld together a moment before adding jojoba carrier oil to the neck of the bottle. Seal with the roller ball. Label and date your perfume. Use on pulse points of the wrist, behind the ears, and/or on the sternum (breastbone) and/or upon the crown of the head. This is potent and you'll only need a small amount on your skin.

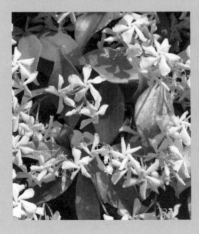
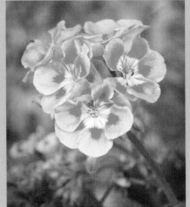
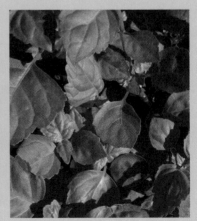

**Part of plant used for essential oils:** Flowers (Technically an absolute, not an essential oil, due to the extraction process by enfleurage. Jasmine's petals are too delicate for distillation.)

**Countries of origin:** India, China, and Persia

**Action:** Antidepressant, aphrodisiac, calms the nervous system, sexual tonic, stimulant

**Uses:**

- *Physically:* Acts as a gentle warming agent to the system as a whole unit, unlike a localized rubefacient. Also used to assist in production of milk for lactating mothers. Relaxes stiffness in muscles and increases circulation in peripheral limbs, but so expensive that black pepper might be a better match for blends with this specific need in mind. Blend with lavender, sweet orange, or neroli for a deep, restful night of sleep. Has also been used to soothe coughs and for throat issues such as hoarseness and laryngitis.
- *Mentally:* Can help the mind relax its whirl of thoughts by inducing a state of calmness.
- *Emotionally:* Add to blends or use for a slow, deep inhalation when anxiety is near or present. Can help reduce stress, nervousness, restlessness, and depression, or when you feel an extreme of hot, cold, or too much or too little of energy within you. Especially beneficial when emotions are so great that you are not in touch with your body. As these blossoms are at their peak—both physically and aromatically—at night, their scent often is used in perfumery to entice the quality of sexiness and sexual confidence, and their oil helps relieve either frozen or heated emotions that stop your connections with your own sexuality or intimacy with others.
- *Spiritually:* When emotions are feeling heavy and overwhelming, can assist in lightening the weight and bringing you to the present. Sometimes we cannot find ourselves until we find the edges of our world and move beyond to explore, creating health and happiness. Jasmine can help you tap into the expansiveness of your intuitive mind and release of internal restraint holding you back from a life of potential and sensitivity.

**Blends well with:** Jasmine is quite potent and can be used on its own (just a single drop will connect with you); however, blends with bergamot, chamomile, frankincense, ginger, grapefruit, lavender, lemon, lemongrass, mandarin, neroli, palmarosa, palo santo, patchouli, rose geranium, rose, sandalwood, sweet orange, vetiver, ylang-ylang

**Precautions:** Use with care: jasmine is expensive and potent. You will not need more than one or two drops per ounce in most blends. It can be overpowering, and in some sensitive individuals can cause headaches if too much is used or applied (rinse off or get fresh air). Generally nonirritant, but can be dermal sensitizing in some individuals.

**Shelf life:** 4 to 5 years

# Lavender

*Cooling—Harmonizing—Vitality*

**Common names:** Lavender, true lavender, English lavender, lavender vera

**Latin name:** *Lavandula angustifolia*

**Botanical family:** Lamiaceae, often referred to as the mint family, a group of herbs and small shrubs that includes patchouli, melissa, mint, basil, rosemary, and thyme. Most originated in the Mediterranean, but these plants are now found around the world, many grown in culinary and home gardens.

**Attributes:** Lavender whispers, soothes, cools, heals, relaxes, and encourages.

**Character:** Has gray-green leaves and dainty purple blooms. Its gentle, soft floral aroma has immediately relaxing effects. Several cousins, *L. spica* (spike lavender) and *L. stoechas* (Spanish lavender), also used for essential oils, have slightly different qualities and uses. The word *lavender* is derived from Latin *lavare* ("to wash") as this herb was often

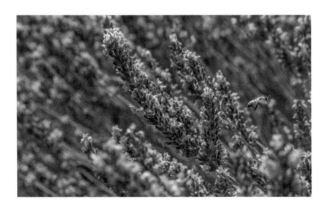

added to water used for laundering. Gentle enough for all ages (use as hydrosols for young ones), and can be used on occasion for anything from bug bites or stings to acne to burns or wound healing (always dilute to avoid any future sensitization). Considered the number one, most versatile essential oil to have for home and professional use, including perfumery, and the best oil for beginners to start with. Can be used in a linen spray, in insect repellents, and for gentle room fresheners, or to breathe a relaxing aroma at the end of the day.

**Unique aroma:** Soft, floral, fresh, velvety, and herbaceous. Both substantial and light, works well as a nice mid note and a harmonizer in blends.

**Aromatic note:** Mid

**Part of plant used for essential oils:** Flowers (although the leaves are scented as well, the flowers are used for distillation)

**Countries of origin:** Native to the Mediterranean; France (especially Provence) is the most famous distillation location, but also distilled in Bulgaria, England, and the United States. There are lavender festivals around the world in summer months.

**Special chemical properties:** High in linalool and linalyl acetate (as much as 40%) that provide harmonization and balancing calm of the body, mind, and spirit.

**Actions:** Analgesic, anti-inflammatory, antifungal, antispasmodic, calms nervous system, lowers blood pressure, reduces anxiety and sensations of pain, sedative, wound healing

**Uses:**

- *Physically:* Can help skin issues such as wounds, cuts, bruises, soft tissue trauma, dry or oily skin, dermatitis, eczema, psoriasis, burns or sunburn, itching, or poorly healing skin. Add to blends to soothe joint or muscle aches and pains, sprains, and stiffness. Add to a diffuser blend for throat infections, coughs, and bronchitis. Add to a blend or use on its own for cramps, colic, flatulence, nausea, irritable bowel syndrome, or emotional nervousness in the stomach. Especially helpful before, during, and after labor for reducing the pain of contractions, and for postpartum perineal recovery as well as with discomforts of PMS, including abdominal cramps. Inhaling this scent greatly reduces pain sensations, often reducing the amount of pain medications needed, and can help lower blood pressure, heart rate, and skin temperature, thus creating a whole body relaxant response.
- *Mentally:* Calm mind, calm body. By clearing away pain sensations and overwhelming emotions, lavender can help your mind relax, which can lead to a fresher outlook on life and access to optimistic possibilities.
- *Emotionally:* Emotions involving heat, anger, and frustration as well as worry, nervous tension, fear, overconcern, or hyper responses, insecurity, and lack of confidence are soothed and smoothed by lavender's calming aroma; use for emotional abuse, trauma, or hormone-induced

### Stress Relief Blend

Add to a personal inhaler and use as needed to calm and reduce pain:

8 to 9 drops lavender
5 to 6 drops sweet orange

emotional ups and downs as well, to sand the rough edges of your feelings and remind you of the softness of your heart. Use alone or add to blends designed for states of moderate sadness and depression; combine with citrus and rose-scented oils for this purpose. Calms the emotional nervous system as a whole.

- *Spiritually:* Lavender whispers to the edges of all levels of your being, "Peacefulness is available to you." By helping restore the central nervous system's natural harmony, it gives the spirit a chance to participate with the experience of humanity.

**Blends well with:** Compatible with just about every available essential oil: bergamot, cedarwood, chamomiles, clary sage, fir, frankincense, geranium, ginger, jasmine, other lavenders, laurel, lemon, lemongrass, mandarin, marjoram, neroli, palmarosa, palo santo, patchouli, peppermint, pine, rose, sandalwood, spruce, sweet orange, vetiver, ylang-ylang

**Precautions:** Although it is the most popular scent worldwide, some will not find lavender to their liking. Whenever you are not interested in an oil, be mindful to follow that indicator; for example, asthmatics and those with allergies, such as hay fever, may not be attracted to lavender. Others may find lavender triggers headaches.

**Shelf life:** 2 to 4 years. Best stored in the refrigerator; can add a drop of vitamin E oil to slow oxidation.

# Sweet Marjoram
*Harmonizer—Centering—Tonifying*

**Common names:** Sweet marjoram, marjoram

**Latin name:** *Origanum marjorana*

**Botanical family:** Lamiaceae, also known as the mint family, a group of herbs and small shrubs that include lavender, patchouli, melissa, mint, basil, rosemary, and thyme. Often grown in culinary and home gardens.

**Attributes:** Marjoram is a bridge between the place

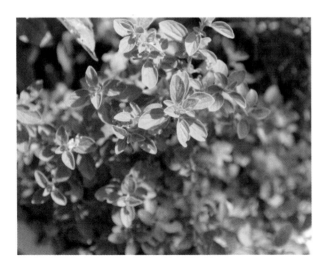

you think you want to go and the place where you are the most harmonized (this scent can help you get past your head). Comforting, warm, analgesic to the body and mind.

**Character:** An aromatic herb that was cultivated by Egyptians, Greeks, and Romans; used in the Middle Ages as medicine; and in more recent history to flavor ale. Grows to 20 to 30 inches in height, with small, dark green, oval leaves and blooms that spike upward in white to pink petals. Prefers warmth over higher-altitude coolness. Has been used as an aromatic plant signifying fertility, love, loyalty, and peace, and as crowns upon newlyweds and at funerals.

**Unique aroma:** Spicy, herbaceous, dry, sharp, penetrating, sweet, slightly woody, warm, camphoraceous

**Aromatic note:** Mid

**Part of plant used for essential oils:** Flowering tops, along with leaves and stems

**Countries of origin:** Believed to have originated in Cypress; flourishes in the Mediterranean, France, Germany, Egypt, and North Africa.

**Actions:** Analgesic, anaphrodisiac (reduces sexual desire), antibacterial, antifungal, antiseptic, antispasmodic, calms nervous system, digestive stimulant, sedative, lowers blood pressure, vasodilator, wound healing

**Uses:**

- *Physically:* An extremely effective and powerful antibacterial, can be added to blends used topically as well as in room diffusers or personal diffusers, to help the body fight off airborne pathogens and viral infections. Quells coughs.

## Muscle Relief Blend

Add to a 1-ounce bottle, swirl the synergy, then top with your choice of carrier oil (jojoba, coconut, almond, or sesame are good starters):

3 drops marjoram

3 drops *Eucalyptus radiata*

3 drops cypress

3 drops ginger

Reduces joint and rheumatic discomfort and swelling as well as growing pains in teenagers. Relieves muscle stiffness, tendonitis, sciatica, spasms, cramps from overexertion or depletion, and menstrual cramps. Use in a tonic rubbed on the abdomen for upset digestion and gas.

- *Mentally:* When the mind spins into overthinking mode and stiffens up in thoughts, unbending, obsessive, not allowing nourishment to enter to feed healthy thoughts, add to your blend or simply inhale the aroma (breathe through the nose, to ignite the parasympathetic "relax and rejuvenate" nervous system). This will help focus and uplift the thoughts within the mind. Obsessive sexual thoughts might be lessened through its anaphrodisiac properties.
- *Emotionally:* Silences the buzz of anxiety, nervous tension, and stress while nourishing the creativity of the heart. Sweet marjoram's uplifting properties are known for shifting lethargy of the body and emotions. Use in times of extreme emotive-thought connections of loss, and deep grief that feels unrelenting, as well as in times signaled by lots of sighing and melancholy to entice the warmth of positive emotions to circulate, clearing stuckness or lack of connections between the mind, heart, and body.
- *Spiritually:* Consider marjoram a comfort for the spirit, a warm heater on a cold day, a hug of self-care, or the view from the mountainside on a spring day. Its feel-good, nurturing energy can calm doubts and bring stability.

**Blends well with:** Bergamot, black pepper, cedarwood, chamomiles, clary sage, cypress, eucalyptus, fir, geranium, helichrysum, juniper berry, lavender, lemongrass, mandarin, melissa, niaouli, palo santo, pine, rosemary, spruce, sweet orange, tea tree. One of the best blend harmonizers. If you are finding that your blend is "almost there" but isn't quite synergizing, add one drop of this oil (more could overpower your blend), or try lavender or sandalwood.

**Precautions:** Always dilute, as too much can cause dermatitis. There are opposing viewpoints as to whether marjoram should be avoided during pregnancy as it is listed as *possibly unsafe* . . . err on the side of caution. Marjoram has GRAS status and is considered safe with normal usage.

**Shelf life:** 3 to 4 years

# Neroli

*Calming—Uplifting—Softening*

**Common names:** Neroli, orange blossom

**Latin name:** *Citrus aurantium* var. *amara*

**Botanical family:** Rutaceae, also known as the citrus family, which includes orange, mandarin, lemon, grapefruit, and clementine. These flowering plants, woody shrubs, and trees are found throughout the warmer temperate regions on the planet.

**Attributes:** Soft around the edges, but deeply penetrating.

**Character:** One of the more expensive essential oils (it takes 1,000 pounds of blossoms to produce just 16 ounces of oil!), neroli comes from the white blooms of the bitter Seville orange tree, plucked in early spring, when they are just opening. Warm, sunny days are best for harvesting; cool, humid days produce an inferior oil. Distillation requires patience and attentiveness to ensure a high-quality oil. Two other essential oils are produced from the same tree: petitgrain is from the tree's leaves and twigs; bitter orange is from the rind of the fruit. Neroli is often adulterated with less expensive oils, such as petitgrain. While neroli can be used interchangeably with petitgrain (which has a "greener" scent), the two are not equals, hence neroli's value therapeutically and financially. It has a distinct aroma and specific attributes. Became widely known after seventeenth-century Italian princess Anne-Maria de la Trémoille of Nerola used this scent as her perfume of choice.

**Unique aroma:** Floral, bittersweet, sweet-turpentine,

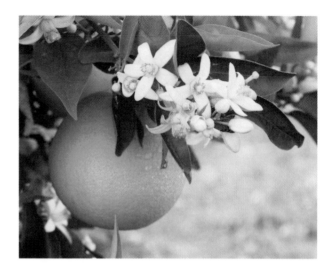

orangelike but softer, powdery, citruslike, warm, hints of honey and spice, heady, rich, underlying green note (even more so if distilled with a few stray leaves and twigs)

**Aromatic note:** Top

**Part of plant used for essential oils:** Flowers

**Countries of origin:** Native to South Asia and India; known throughout the Mediterranean, now distilled mostly in France, as well as in Italy and Tunisia, but grown in temperate regions across the globe, including the United States and South America.

**Actions:** Antidepressant, antifungal, anti-inflammatory, antimicrobial, antioxidant, antiparasitic, antiseptic, aphrodisiac, calms, digestive, nervous system stimulant, sedative, and tonic

**Uses:**

- *Physically:* In skin ointments, used for antiaging and assisting in areas of fine wrinkles, while harmonizing excess or deficient oil production on the skin. Use for acne, reducing scarring, and areas that may need extra regenerative support, such as wound healing and scars. Helps regulate blood pressure and calm the central nervous system, which can redirect energy from pain sensations toward healing. Add to blends designed to relieve muscle and joint pains and cramping, including menstrual pain, and abdominal spasms, flatulence, and colic. Frequently used for sedative, relaxing purposes as well as in aphrodisiac blends (historically added to brides' bouquets and hair for this purpose).

- *Mentally:* Boosts thinking positively, and a good addition to synergies designed for those with disconnections between their body and mind (use with patchouli to assist with this).
- *Emotionally:* When thoughts are connected to deeply hidden or unsurfaced emotions, neroli can melt such resistance by encouraging self-confidence and reassurance. Sensuality and emotion are part of the human experience, and intimately connected to the limbic system. This oil gently awakens the connection between the pleasures of sight, smell, feel, touch, and thought. Use for anxiety and grief.
- *Spiritually:* Can help you find focus and beauty in the small and wonderful.

**Blends well with:** Bergamot, bitter orange, cedarwood, clary sage, frankincense, geranium, grapefruit, helichrysum, lavender, lemon, marjoram,

## Face Oil Blend

Add to a 1-ounce amber or cobalt blue glass bottle, then top with a 50/50 blend of rosehip and apricot seed carrier oils:

3 drops neroli
3 drops lavender
1 to 2 drops rose geranium
2 to 3 drops helichrysum

Keep your total drops to 10 to maintain safe levels for the face. Store in the refrigerator to maintain rosehip's delicate nature.

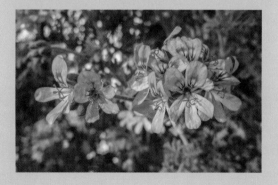

melissa, palmarosa, palo santo, petitgrain, pine, rose, rosemary, sandalwood, sweet orange

**Precautions:** Always dilute; neroli is so precious, you'll want to make sure you get the most out of its properties. It is also potent, so a little goes a long way. Nonirritant and nonphotosensitive. Petitgrain is an option when not available.

**Shelf life:** 4 to 5 years

# Rose

*Self-love—Heart—Love*

**Common names:** Rose, damask rose

**Latin names:** *Rosa damascena*; (white rose) *Rosa damascena* var. *alba*

**Botanical family:** Lamiaceae, the family of roses, which includes apricot and almond (both used for carrier oils) as well as strawberries and raspberries. As a family, grown all over the world, but prefers northern temperate areas.

**Special qualities:** The essential oil equivalent of the seed of love. A small drop holds the potential of an entire universe expressing love. Powerful, gentle, intoxicating, healing and wonderful. Dubbed the "queen of flowers" by poet Sappho in 600 BC.

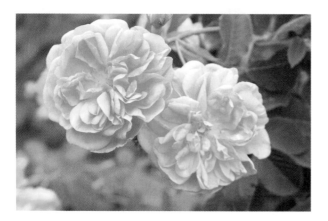

**Character:** Cultivated, beloved, and honored in China, Persia, India, ancient Rome and Greece, as well as in Arab cultures. The essential oil was first discovered in 1582 in Persia when Emperor Djihanguyr and Princess Nour-Dijhan were rowing through a canal filled with rose water at their wedding feast. The sun had gently heated the waters, creating separation of the essential oil, which had risen to the top, appearing as a film. The essential oil was skimmed off the top to use as a natural perfume. Otto of roses was developed from this discovery. However, it was Persian alchemist Avicenna who distilled the first essential oil—rose! To date, this comes in two forms: a true essential oil, from Bulgaria, known as rose otto, and an absolute from France, known as rose absolute. It takes 60,000 roses to distill a single ounce of rose otto. Perfumery often uses the absolute form due to its lower cost, but this form has possibilities of contamination by solvents used in this extraction method.

**Unique aroma:** Deeply floral, soft, sweet, honeylike, rich, warm, feminine, potent, astringent

**Aromatic note:** Mid

**Part of plant used for essential oils:** Petals; must be picked before dawn. The light of the sun opens the stomata of the petals, releasing their fragrance. It is the only way to capture their aroma intact.

**Countries of origin:** Asia, originally. Bulgaria's Valley of Roses is thought to have had *R. damascena* brought from Tunisia in 1420. For centuries prior, though, it already held a place with Turkish empires. Distilled in Bulgaria, as well as in Morocco, Turkey, and India.

**Special chemical properties:** Contains 275 components. Its greatest chemical is citronellol (70%), but what sets a rose's aroma apart is its small amounts of beta-damascenone (0.14%) and beta-ionon (0.03%), discovered in the 1960s and '70s, which are solely responsible for the distinct, potent aroma of rose (Crow 2016).

**Actions:** Antibacterial, antidepressant, anti-infectious, anti-inflammatory, antiseptic, antiviral, aphrodisiac, astringent, calms the nervous system, reduces anxiety, sedative, sexual, general and uterine tonic, wound healing

**Uses:**

- *Physically:* Add to skin care or facial oils as a harmonizer for sebum production and cellular regeneration, to assist with acne and mature skin, but especially for dry, infected, and sensitive skin. Soothes eczema, rashes, dermatitis, and skin that needs system support to repair; supports broken capillaries, lymphatic drainage, and circulation in general. Also used in hair products. Regulates menstruation and assists with menopause, ovary concerns, and postnatal depression. Also, rose hydrosol (rose water) can be used as a face toner spray before facial oils; to cool the mind, heart, and body, and as a compress for fevers; for teething; for minor scrapes, in mouthwashes, to mist the air; as well as a safe wash for vaginitis.
- *Mentally:* Supports beneficial, positive

---

## Face Oil Divine

Add to a ½-ounce carrier of rosehip oil:

1 drop rose
1 drop jasmine
1 drop sandalwood
1 drop helichrysum

Apply 1 to 2 drops of the blend on a clean face (after spraying with rose otto hydrosol) in a light dabbing motion rather than rubbing the skin. Use in the morning and before bed on a clean face. Store in the refrigerator to support rosehip's vitality.

---

thoughts, and therefore emotional well-being (see next use).

- *Emotionally:* Emotions are said to begin in the mind. As they are so connected, harmonization of mind and heart are by far rose's greatest effect. Soothes and cools nervous tension and feelings of stress, stabilizes mood swings, and allows for easier coping and clearer decision making. During deep emotions of grief and loss, depression, and despair, gently opens the heart to loving once again. Can allay sexual hesitations, frigidity, or nervousness, and can be added to aphrodisiac synergies and blends. Nurtures all heart-related experiences of love, beauty, and peace. Connects the thinking mind to observe and the sensitive heart to feel these attributes within oneself, promoting self-love that overflows in trickles and waves to others.

- *Spiritually:* Encourages feeling more love and compassion for yourself, taking care and allowing tenderness to be part of your world; those waves of kindness roll outward to meet the world, which responds in turn.

**Blends well with:** Cardamom, clary sage, cypress, frankincense, grapefruit, jasmine, lavender, lemon, mandarin, neroli, palo santo, patchouli, rose geranium, sandalwood, sweet orange, vanilla, vetiver, ylang-ylang. For skin repair, add to blends with helichrysum.

**Precautions:** The most expensive essential oil on the market, each drop costing several dollars apiece. If you are unable to have this essential oil in your collection (and really there is no substitute), do take into consideration that palmarosa and rose geranium have *some* similar aromatic benefits; read their attributes and precautions and see whether they may suit your needs.

**Shelf life:** 4 to 5 years

# Ylang-ylang

*Sweet—Exotic—Soothing*

**Common names:** Ylang-ylang, derived from the Filipino word *alang-ilang* ("fluttering in the breeze"); also known as the "flower of flowers" and "poor man's jasmine"

**Latin name:** *Cananga odorata*

**Botanical family:** Annonceae, also known as the custard apple family, encompassing 130 genera and 2,300 species of tropical and subtropical fragrant trees, shrubs, and climbers, with evergreen leaves and resins and fruits. Ylang-ylang is the only essential oil in the family that is commonly used in aromatherapy.

**Attributes:** Fragrant, protective, seducing, soothing, and calming.

**Character:** Often found in tropical islands and forests, usually as a small tree (up to 60 feet high), but can grow taller in the right environmental conditions. Some cousins have similar blooms, but ylang-ylang's yellow flowers produce the most fragrance. The blossoms are picked, like rose petals, just before dawn. Unlike rose, though, ylang-ylang releases its aroma through the night, from dusk to dawn, to attract the night moths that pollinate its flowers. Propagated from seed, plants grow very quickly, but their blooms are picked three to four years into their growth cycle for a more mature fragrance. Used for lei-like ornamentation in the Philippines, and known there in legend as the name of a girl, Ylang, who vanished into thin air when a man dared to touch her arm as he proposed marriage; he is said to still wander the garden looking for her, calling her name: "Ylang, Ylang." This oil is one of the secret ingredients, along with rose and jasmine, in the famous perfume Chanel No. 5.

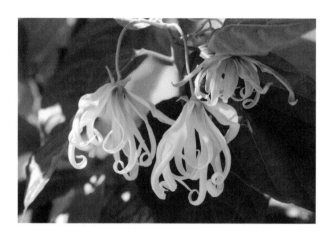

**Unique aroma:** Warm, sweet, heavy, heady, sensual, exotic, balsamic, slightly spicy, tenacious, penetrating, tropical, slightly fruity, and slightly spicy

**Aromatic note:** Mid to base

**Part of plant used for essential oils:** Flowers

**Countries of origin:** Native to Malaysia and Indonesia; also found in the Philippines, Java, Sumatra, Madagascar, Australia, Thailand, and Vietnam. Has been grown in Florida, in the United States, but does not reach the same heights as in its native lands.

**Special chemical properties:** This oil's distillation phases affect its chemistry. Its top distillations, Extra Superior or Extra, containing the most esters, which are its most volatile components, are considered the finest and most refined grades. The First, Second, and Third grades have fewer esters, and so the slower-vaporizing sesquiterpenes cause the aroma to become deeper and richer. "Complete" distillations are a blend of all the distillation stages. Unless you are looking for specific chemical compounds, using "Ylang-ylang Complete" is perfect (and less costly than Extra).

**Actions:** Antidepressant, anti-inflammatory, antiparasitic, antispasmodic, aphrodisiac, calms the nervous system and lowers blood pressure, sexual tonic

**Uses:**

- *Physically:* Systemically, helps cool and slow down the effects of stress on the heart, such as high blood pressure and heart palpitations, by clearing excess heat, as well as produces general deep calm within the body, including the mind and emotions. Use in abdominal massage may ease menstrual tensions and muscular cramps as well as assist in the regulation of menstruation. Has been used for support in diabetic and to allay epileptic concerns (inhaled before a seizure). Use in hair tonics and scalp massages; historically thought to prevent hair loss. Can be added to facial oils and creams for regulation of excess or deficient sebum of the skin.

- *Mentally:* Agitated minds create agitated hearts. Cooling and soothing the mind, relaxing the thoughts, benefits the body; ylang-ylang can assist in smoothing away long-held stress and post-traumatic memories by allowing them to be processed and released. Thoughts that lock down from past experiences tend to roll over into emotional blocks. Clearing these blocks can

## Meditation Blend
### (diffuser)

Add the following to a room water diffuser:

1 drop ylang-ylang
1 drop patchouli

These are both penetrating scents; it will not take many drops to fill the air. Always start a low drop count, you can always add more, but cannot take it away.

open the mind, heart, and body to better communicate with one another.

- *Emotionally:* Like rose and jasmine, can guide the heart to a place of coolness, calmness, kindness, and self-love. Relaxing and uplifting, ylang-ylang promotes positive feelings, joy, and peace as well as nurtures creativity and self-assurance. Producing euphoric moods, romantic openness, and inner trust, opens the heart to the possibility of confidence in relationships, sensuality, sexuality, gentleness, and tenderness. Nervous tensions, feelings of isolation, and separation are softened and melted away.
- *Spiritually:* Adding a drop or two to blends along with a drop of soft vanilla absolute, rose otto, and sandalwood might make quite a lasting impression throughout your day. Euphoric spaces held for contemplative peaceful moments will benefit from a drop of this essential oil, along with palo santo, frankincense, sandalwood, sweet orange, and vetiver.

**Blends well with:** Bergamot, frankincense, helichrysum, jasmine, lavender, neroli, palo santo, patchouli, rose geranium, rose, sandalwood, sweet orange, vanilla, vetiver

**Precautions:** Always dilute. Very potent, use no more than 1 to 2 drops per ounce of carrier in a synergistic blend. If the scent seems too strong, try in a more highly diluted blend or personal inhaler. Too much of this odor can create headaches for some, so be mindful—less is more. You may also even consider doing inhalations in highly diluted forms.

**Shelf life:** 4 to 5 years

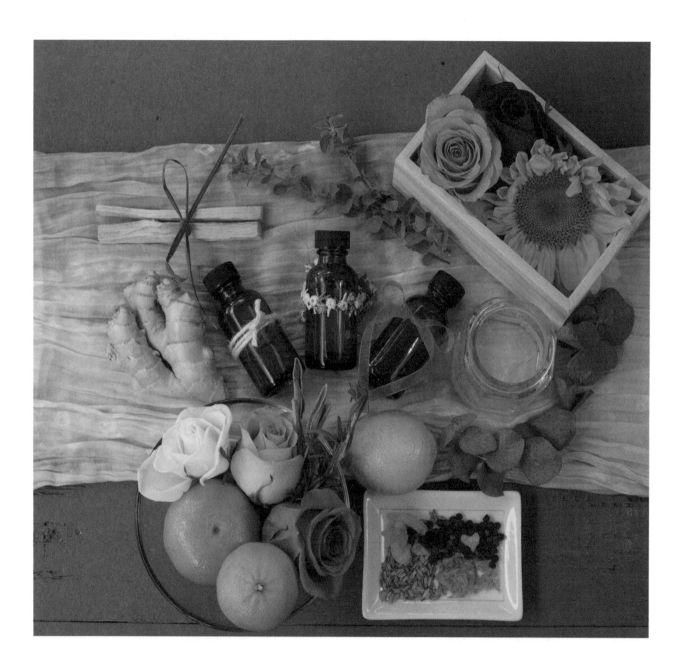

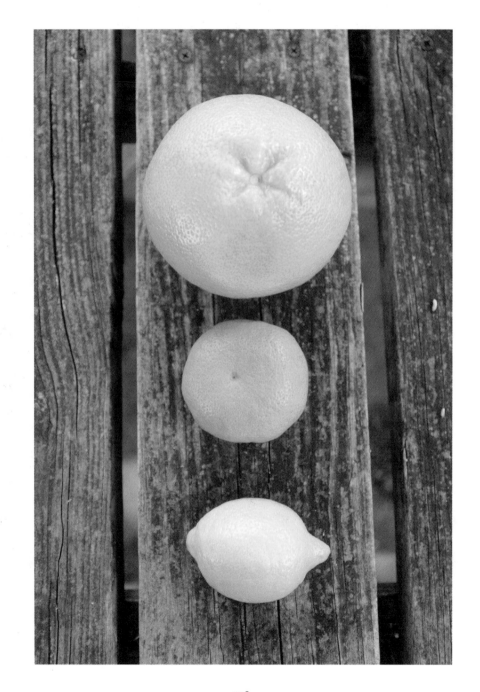

# CHAPTER 11

# Rinds and Fruits

*A table, a chair, a bowl of fruit, and a violin; what else does a man need to be happy?* —Albert Einstein

## Joy—Lightness—Protection

Rinds and fruits invoke joyful creativity, lead one part of oneself to another part, protect until it is no longer needed and then the next stage can naturally occur ("This, too, shall pass"), and teach mindfulness, lightness, and sweetness in life. Fruit brings sunny dispositions, the freshness and juiciness that life embodies. Fruits and rinds also have a calming effect on the nervous system as well as uplift and dispel heavy emotions and thoughts. Citrus also clears the air of stagnant or stale feelings.

Enzymes held within fruit and the rinds of citrus are designed to ensure ripeness, its full potential. Once achieved, the seeds it contains must be released somehow and the original outer protection is softened. The seeds are released by consumption or by the plants letting them go. Citrus is easily bruised or damaged, therefore a certain mindfulness must be present when holding fruit and working with its essence. Fruit is only available for a season, a reminder that heaviness is a fleeting moment, as is happiness, but experiences in the moment can be treasured.

Note that juniper berry, included in this chapter, is not citrus.

Phototoxicity is a concern for some citrus. If in doubt, save it for the diffuser or personal inhaler, but with a little care, you can learn how to safely use citrus in home remedies. Observe all the safety precautions listed to avoid flying "too close to the sun" with these sunshiny essential oils.

### CITRUS PHOTOTOXICITY

*Do not use* in topical applications 12 to 24 hours prior to exposure to sunlight, UV light exposure, or

**PHOTOTOXIC**

Bergamot (cold pressed), *Citrus bergamia*
Bitter orange (cold pressed), *Citrus aurantium*
Grapefruit (cold pressed and distilled), *Citrus paradisi*—
low risk—use under 4%
Lemon (cold pressed), *Citrus limon*
Lime (cold pressed), *Citrus medica*

**NONPHOTOTOXIC**

Bergamot FCF (FCF has the bergaptene/furanocoumarins
removed), *Citrus bergamia*
Bergamot (steam distilled), *Citrus bergamia*
Lemon (steam distilled), *Citrus limon*
Lime (steam distilled), *Citrus medica*
Mandarin/tangerine (cold pressed or steam distilled),
*Citrus reticulata*
Sweet orange (cold pressed or steam distilled), *Citrus
sinensis*

using a tanning bed. Severe burns can occur. Some citrus oils absorb UV light without causing sensations of the burn until it is too late.

If you cannot remember which oils are phototoxic, then assume what you have is phototoxic. It is much safer to assume safety precautions are necessary than think they are not. The risk to you and your family is not worth the gamble. Until you are intimately familiar with nontoxic citrus, assume they are all phototoxic for your blending purposes.

Robert Tisserand and Rodney Young's book *Essential Oil Safety,* 2nd edition, includes a full list of essential oils considered to be phototoxic. Only

citrus-related essential oils profiled in this book are listed here.

# Bergamot
*Encouraging—Uplifting—Relaxing*
**Common name:** Bergamot (French pronunciation has a silent t)
**Latin name:** *Citrus bergamia*
**Botanical family:** Rutaceae, primarily shrubs and trees and some herbs, commonly called the citrus family due to the high level of fruit-bearing citrus trees; also called the rue family. The family comprises 160 genera and more than 2,000 species; the majority grow in warm, temperate, or tropical regions.
**Attributes:** Encouraging to those who need to remember what ease feels like on all levels of being. Considered one of the best essential oils for uplifting the mind and emotions, and relieving anxiety, when used safely. Can be sedating or stimulating, depending on the blend.
**Character:** A flowering tree growing to 16 feet tall, with fragrant star-shaped white flowers and dark green ovate leaves, a cross between bitter orange and lemon. The essential oil is green or olive green, but changes to yellow when air or age have oxidized. Christopher Columbus imported bergamot from the Canary Islands to Spain and then to Italy. Used medicinally in Italy since the 1700s; however, its medicinal uses predate this; has long been used in Ayurveda to calm heightened nervous states (Vata) and in Traditional Chinese Medicine, especially with liver or stagnant qi. One of the ingredients in

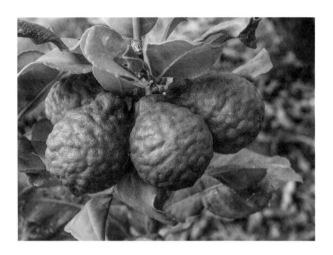

Hungary water, used since ancient times for paralysis and the complexion. Has many uses, from antiseptics to being a fixative in perfumes; bergamot pulp is used to make citric acid, and its leaves create the unique aroma and scent of Earl Grey tea. (Do not confuse this plant with monarda, also known as bee balm, a common herb also referred to as bergamot.)

**Unique aroma:** Refreshing, uplifting, citrusy, sweet-fruity, rich, sharp, exotic, fresh, spicy, floral, slightly green

**Aromatic note:** Top

**Part of plant used for essential oils:** Expressed from the fresh peel or zest of the fruit

**Countries of origin:** Originally from tropical Asia, now grown in southern Italy, primarily Calabria.

**Special chemical properties:** High in limonene (46%), linalyl acetate (26%), and linalool (6%), all known for calming.

**Actions:** Air purifier, antibacterial, antidepressant, antifungal, anti-inflammatory, antiviral, calming, deodorant, digestive regulating (under- or overeating), reduces anxiety, sedative, tonic, wound healing

**Uses:**

- *Physically:* Due to its phototoxicity potential, care must be used when bergamot is applied topically; see Precautions. However, in safe dilutions and applications, can act as powerful antiseptic for acne, herpes, psoriasis, ulcers, wounds, as well as harmonize sebum in oily hair and skin. Also has a connection to regulating appetite (caution: never ingest). When inhaled as a scent, can help abate flatulence, nervous indigestion, and nausea; also, for digestive concerns, add to a blend containing fennel, chamomile, and ginger and massage clockwise on the abdomen. If you have been diagnosed with vaginal pruritus or a gonococcal infection, you may find some relief by using bergamot in a bath at a 0.5% dilution (but always ask your doctor before doing so) (Price 1995 [1988]).

- *Mentally:* If your thoughts tend to move into a rut or routinely reset to negativity, or you have a hard time changing old patterns or even finding the motivation to want to change, bergamot can help you see and pursue shifts as a new opportunity. (Small changes can have big impacts!)

- *Emotionally:* Incredibly beneficial used as an aroma in the air. Can aid anxiety, depression, mood swings (hormone-induced and otherwise), or stuck emotions. When outbreaks of acne, hives, and eczema are worsened by high levels

## Sleep Diffuser Blend

Add to a water room diffuser 30 minutes before going to bed:

**1 to 2 drops bergamot**
**1 to 2 drops lavender**

Turn off the diffuser when you go to bed.

Alternatively, drop a drop or two of each oils on a cotton ball and place bedside throughout the night. (Place the cotton ball in a glass or ceramic bowl, not plastic, metal, or wood.)

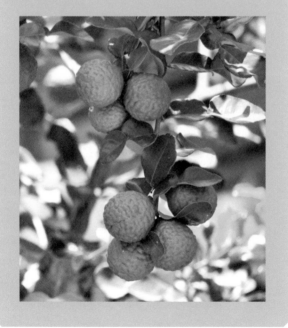

of anxiety, can soothe the connection between the heart and mind (thus the body benefits). Can help regulate mood swings of PMS and menopause. Apply a soothing massage blend of bergamot, clary sage, and lavender to the abdomen (avoiding sunlight or UV rays to this area for 12 to 24 hours after application). Those with insomnia, depression, and anxiety will find this a wonderful oil to diffuse 30 minutes before going to bed (turn off the diffuser once in bed).

- *Spiritually:* Ayurveda describes a state in which you are out of harmony with your true nature as something that can be adjusted by bringing all parts of the whole in connection with one another. To treat the mind or body only, ignoring the spirit, is incomplete. This essential oil helps to connect all systems, uplifting the spirit, reducing stress in the emotional heart and mind, and supporting the body. Add to your meditative blends when you wish to bring the sunshine into your contemplative space (both to warm and awaken as well as to soothe and soften).

**Blends well with:** Angelica root, chamomile, coriander, clary sage, cypress, eucalyptus, frankincense, ho wood, jasmine, juniper, lemon, lemongrass, lime, lavender, mandarin, neroli, peppermint, rose geranium, rosemary, sweet orange, vetiver, ylang-ylang

**Precautions:** *Highly phototoxic.* Keep dilution ratio to 0.4% or less (2 to 3 drops per ounce of carrier oil). Photosensitivity of skin is increased due to the presence of the compound bergapten. Best used as a scent to inhale in the day or to use topically in early evening or night, to ensure time away from the sun's rays. Use with care on skin and always dilute, as this essential oil can cause pigmentation. If used in essential oil jewelry, do not allow the oil to touch the skin and do not wear in direct sunlight. Avoid old and oxidized oils. Store all citrus oils in dark containers; refrigeration is recommended.

**Note:** The essential oil bergamot FCF (furanocoumarin-free), sometimes called rectified bergamot, has been stripped of its photosensitizing components, which allows it to be used without the risk of phototoxicity. Order from a reputable supplier. Unless it is listed as bergamot FCF, always assume it is phototoxic and use all appropriate safety guidelines.

**Shelf life:** 1 to 3 years

# Grapefruit

*Enlighten—Satisfy—Cleanse*

**Common name:** Grapefruit

**Latin name:** *Citrus x paradisi*

**Botanical family:** Rutaceae, primarily shrubs and trees and some herbs, commonly called the citrus family due to the high level of fruit-bearing citrus trees; also called the rue family. The family comprises 160 genera and more than 2,000 species; the majority grow in warm, temperate, or tropical regions.

**Attributes:** A promoter of lightness, uplifts and satisfies the mind-body connection.

**Character:** Grapefruit is a cross between pomelo (*C. grandis*) and sweet orange (*C. sinensis*). Its trees stand 20 to 30 feet tall, with large, glossy green leaves and fragrant white flowers. Its common name came from the visual growth of its botanical fruit, bunched together like large grapes. Its Latin name, meaning "paradise," celebrates its discovery in Jamaica in the 1600s. The botanical fruit is harvested in late spring to early or midsummer. It is eaten for its high vitamin C content; its essential oils are used in cosmetics, flavoring, soaps, and perfumes as well as in therapeutic aromatherapy. Used in Ayurveda and Traditional Chinese Medicine, grapefruit is said to reduce stagnant energy in the body.

**Unique aroma:** Fresh, citrusy, sweet, sweet-bitter, light, zing, acidic

**Aromatic note:** Top

**Part of plant used for essential oils:** Peel of the fruit, cold expressed (occasionally distilled)

**Countries of origin:** Malaysia and Southeast Asia; also found in Jamaica. The United States produces the most essential oil, in Florida and California.

**Special chemical properties:** Highest chemical is d-limonene (up to 93%), but it has 0.6% nootkatone, a ketone, which provides its distinctive scent.

**Actions:** Air purifier, antibacterial, antidepressant, antifungal, antimicrobial, antiseptic, antiviral, astringent, detoxifier, disinfectant, lymphatic decongestant, reduces anxiety, stimulates digestion

**Uses:**

- *Physically:* Added to air purification blends, can clear airways and sinus congestion. Use as a facial toner, for stretch marks, to reduce skin

## After Shower/After Workout

Stimulates circulation, soothes muscles, and supports lymphatic movement. Create the following essential oil synergy first in a 1-ounce (amber glass or PET) container, then top with your favorite carrier oil or unscented cream/lotion or carrier oil:

4 drops grapefruit

4 drops cypress

4 drops ginger

Towel dry, then massage onto large muscles of legs, hips, lower back, and abdomen (preferably within 3 minutes of drying off). This dilution contains only 0.5% of grapefruit (4 drops in a 1-ounce carrier), well below the recommended photosensitive suggested range of 4%.

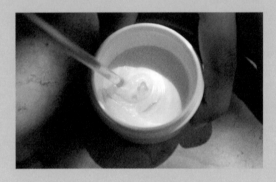

inflammation, and as an astringent for acne and herpes. Add to massage blends for sluggish circulatory, lymphatic (including edema), cellulite, and digestive concerns (e.g., constipation), as well as for muscle aches and pains, rheumatism, and swollen joints holding heat. Although can assist with sleep disorders, such as insomnia, not typically sedating; rather, regulating. PMS discomfort may find reprieve simply by inhalation of this essential oil. Can balance the entire body by reducing emotions that may cause "overindulging in foods and alcohol, especially sweets, chocolate, and biscuits" (Mojay 1997).

- *Mentally:* Calms the mind from thoughts of criticism, especially of oneself (and others), leading to thoughts of positivity and encouragement, rather than those that perpetuate frustrations. Those who feel accustomed or entitled to instant gratification may develop patience with this essential oil.
- *Emotionally:* Can help process and release old frustrations and anger deeply seated in experiences with shame or authoritative misuse of power, perhaps healing and opening up to the inner child within. Eases stress-related feelings, including anxiety and dissatisfaction.
- *Spiritually:* Lightening and enlightening

grapefruit allows for the digestion of ideas, concepts and ways of being (there is another way—you can choose another way), cleansing one of stuck, stagnant, or no longer needed notions and softening impatience to allow the nurturing of the spirit within to take place in stages, as needed and without empty instant reactions.

**Blends well with:** Bergamot, black pepper, clary sage, clove, cypress, frankincense, ginger, jasmine, juniper, lavender, lemon, lime, mandarin, monarda, palo santo, peppermint, rose geranium, sandalwood, Scots pine, sweet orange, ylang-ylang

**Precautions:** Has a low dermal irritant potential of photosensitivity. Topical preparations must be in dilutions of 4% or less (about 30 drops maximum per ounce of carrier). Topical applications above this should assume phototoxic safety protocols and stay out of the sun/UV rays for 12 to 24 hours. Wash-off products (e.g., hand soap) may be used in higher dilutions. Compresses with direct exposure to the skin and as baths, use at 1% or less, diluted with a dispersant to avoid any adverse skin reactions (no more than 7 to 10 drops, diluted, in a full adult bath) (Shutes 2016). Store in dark container; refrigeration recommended. Avoid old or oxidized oils, which can cause skin sensitivity.

**Note:** The common warning against mixing medications with grapefruit refers to components in grapefruit *juice* that are not present in the essential oil (Tisserand and Young 2002).

**Shelf life:** 1 to 2 years

# Lemon

*Invigorate—Open—Possibility*

**Common name:** Lemon

**Latin names:** *Citrus limonum*, also known as *Citrus limon*

**Botanical family:** Rutaceae, primarily shrubs and trees and some herbs, commonly called the citrus family due to the high level of fruit-bearing citrus trees; also called the rue family. The family comprises 160 genera and more than 2,000 species; the majority grow in warm, temperate, or tropical regions.

**Attributes:** Lemon is the sweetness of the sun, ready to start the day. Its scent is clean, fresh, and familiar. People say it makes them smile and open their heart.

**Character:** Like many of its cousins that are similar in size as a small tree, 10 to 20 feet high, lemon can also be a low spreading bush. In common with many of its citrus relatives, it has wonderfully fragrant white flowers. A single tree can produce an astonish-

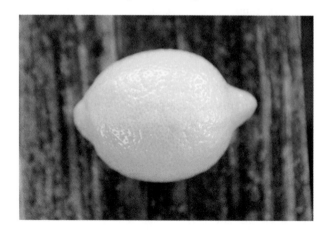

ing 1,500 fruits in a year. The fruit, rich in vitamin C, is used in the food industry for flavoring and juice. Roman and Greek empires have been familiar with its use for scurvy and anemia, and Ayurvedic and Traditional Chinese Medicine protocols used lemon's botanical essences to dry out excess phlegm. In 1698, Nicholas Lemery mentioned the medicinal value of lemon as being a blood cleanser and flatulence reliever (Mojay 1997). Has been used for centuries for concerns of toxicity, boosting immunity and abating infection. Lemon is also used in perfumery.

**Unique aroma:** Sharp, citrus, refreshing, bright, sour, light, slightly sweet

**Aromatic note:** Top

**Part of plant used for essential oils:** Peel of the fruit, expressed

**Countries of origin:** Thought to have originated in India to Italy, then spread throughout Asia and the Mediterranean. The United States is also a major modern producer of this essential oil.

**Special chemical properties:** Contains d-limonene (up to 70%) and $\beta$-pinene (up to 10%).

**Actions:** Antibacterial, anticoagulant, antidepressant, anti-infectious, anti-inflammatory, antiseptic, antiviral, astringent, antioxidant, antimicrobial, digestive stimulant, immunity booster, lymphatic, reduces anxiety

**Uses:**

- *Physically:* In safe dilutions acts as a harmonizer for oily skin and an astringent for insect bites, acne, and boils, and can be used on warts. Soothes tired skin, mature skin, cellulite, and infections (again, properly diluted). Has anticoagulation and astringent properties; cleans and clears out bruises, supports blood flow with varicose veins, broken capillaries, hemorrhoids and nosebleeds, and supports circulation. The same components soothe muscle aches and pains as well as swelling. Digestively, can help sluggish organs that have been overloaded to move food and drink and release stagnant energy; likewise, unblocks the lymphatic system. Used in diffusers and personal inhalers, acts as an antiviral and antifungal air purifier, helpful during times of illness and in rooms where a lot of people have visited (potential for more pathogens). Use for mild headaches.

- *Mentally:* Just as the sun lightens up a room, so does this essential oil assist in bringing focus through inhalation.

- *Emotionally:* Reduces anxiety and calms the emotions and thoughts in the mind. Depression, frustrations, anger, irritation, and overzealousness can be quelled by the lightness of a little lemon in your environment. Inhale this aroma when feelings feel hot and heavy.

- *Spiritually:* Revitalizes the spirit with the energy of the sun, dissipating blocks, opening the heart, soothing the mind, and supporting the body to flow in a gentle, constant motion of self-confidence.

**Blends well with:** Bergamot, cedar, chamomile, cypress, Douglas fir, elemi, *Eucalyptus globulus* or *E. radiata*, fennel, frankincense, geranium, ginger, grapefruit, juniper berry, lavender, lime, mandarin, melissa, niaouli, palmarosa, palo santo, pine, ravintsara, rose, sandalwood, tea tree

**Precautions:** Expressed lemon essential oil is considered to have a dermal toxic potential of photosensitivity. It absorbs UV rays and your skin will burn if you are wearing it and are exposed to the sun or tanning beds (or any UV rays) within 12 to 24 hours of application. Topical preparations must be in dilutions of 2% or less. Wash-off products (e.g., hand soap) may be used in higher dilutions. Compresses with direct exposure to the skin and as baths, use at 1% or less, diluted with a dispersant to avoid any adverse skin reactions (no more than 7 to 10 drops, diluted, in a full adult bath) (Shutes 2016). Store in dark containers; refrigeration recommended. Avoid old or oxidized oils, which can cause skin sensitivity.

**Note:** *Distilled* lemon oil is not considered phototoxic, but can be skin sensitizing if oxidized.

Distilled lemon essential oil is mostly found in the perfumery industry and is considered an inferior oil therapeutically, hence you will not find it very often in aromatherapy.

**Shelf life:** 1 to 2 years

## Mandarin

*Playful—Uplifting—Inviting*

**Common names:** Mandarin, also called tangerine

**Latin name:** *Citrus reticulate*

**Botanical family:** Rutaceae, primarily shrubs and trees and some herbs, commonly called the citrus family due to the high level of fruit-bearing citrus trees; also called the rue family. The family comprises 160 genera and more than 2,000 species; the majority grow in warm, temperate, or tropical regions.

**Attributes:** Playful and versatile, yet soothing; a good beginner citrus oil.

Familiar, light, sweet, and good for the mind, also easing depression and stomach concerns.

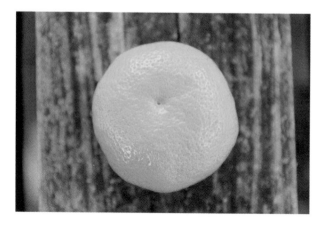

**Character:** As a small tree of only about 13 feet high, mandarin produces small fruits, smaller and sweeter than those of its close cousin, the sweet orange. Grows in warm, humid, and tropical areas. Has been used as food, flavoring, offerings, and gifts. When harvested for essential oils, gives greatest yield as semiripe fruit. This fruit is often called tangerine, because the fruits originally passed through the port of Tangiers on their way to the United States. Tangerines are technically a subset of mandarins—all tangerines are mandarins, but not all mandarins are tangerines! The two do have slightly different aromas. However, you may use the two essential oils interchangeably, although mandarin is considered superior to tangerine.

**Unique aroma:** Sweet, fresh, citrusy, slightly spicy, uplifting, light, tangy

**Aromatic note:** Top

**Part of plant used for essential oils:** Peel, zest, rind, extracted by expression and steam distillation

**Countries of origin:** China, but now includes the United States. Often referred to as mandarin in Europe and tangerine in the United States.

**Special chemical properties:** True tangerines have a higher note limonene content (up to 92%); mandarins contain less (up to 74%) (Tisserand and Young 2014), yet are still considered quite high in content. D-limonene has been said to assist in weight loss and respiratory issues, such as bronchitis.

**Actions:** Analgesic, antidepressant, antiseptic, central nervous system tonic, deodorant, digestive tonic, immunity booster, reduces anxiety and fevers, sedative

**Uses:**

- *Physically:* Used for clockwise abdominal massage (always dilute in a carrier), aids digestive upsets, especially in children, those who are in fragile health, and the elderly. Just smelling this essential oil may stimulate your saliva glands, a sign that it is useful in stimulating both digestion and appetite—try after an illness if you need to replenish your body with food and have not had an appetite. Helps clear congested skin, especially when sebum levels tend to show to be oily on both skin and hair. Also relieves congested areas of cellulite and edema. Add to a lotion or oil for muscle spasms, aches and pains, or stimulating circulation. Diffused in the air, uplifts as well as clears the air environmentally and in bodily airways.

- *Mentally:* Use in your evening relaxing blends or as a morning or midafternoon reset in your diffuser or personal inhaler, or when you need to regain focus with an elevated attitude.

- *Emotionally:* Supports the body and heart when stress- or hormone-induced coping mechanisms falter. Can assist your overall sense of well-being, calming the waves of pendulum mood swings of emotions, such as anger, frustrations, depression, fear, or limited expressions. Especially helpful for reducing anxiety and nervousness, which ultimately helps with sleep (try

# Spicy Citrus Feel-Good Personal Inhaler

Add the following to a personal inhaler, using as needed to find that feel-good boost. Place in an inhaler that can hold between 25 and 30 drops:

5 drops mandarin

5 drops sweet orange

5 drops grapefruit

3 drop patchouli

4 to 5 drops ginger

Label properly.

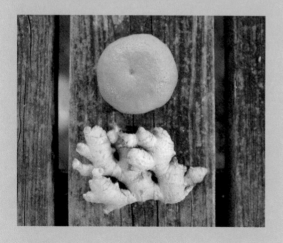

with lavender or neroli for rest) and relationship interactions (try with neroli, laurel, or black pepper for confidence). Also calms heightened activity, such as in children, or overzealousness (Traditional Chinese Medicine calls this excess joy that takes over the system, which can potentially "short out" the nervous system).

- *Spiritually:* Creativity blooms when the mind and heart can connect. Add to a blend with patchouli and fennel in your diffuser for an interesting uplifting creative spark with clear, grounded intentions. Add to a blend containing palo santo to open your intuitive and creative side.

**Blends well with:** Bergamot, cedarwood. chamomile, clary sage, clementine, fennel, frankincense, grapefruit, jasmine, laurel, lavender, lemon, neroli, palmarosa, palo santo, patchouli, rose geranium, rose, sandalwood, sweet orange, vetiver, ylang-ylang

**Precautions:** Always dilute for topical application, to avoid skin irritation. Mandarin is one of the few citrus oils considered to be nonphototoxic and one of the safer and gentlest essential oils for various ages; however, some sources suggest caution with all citrus essential oils applied to the skin, as a general safety guideline (which might be more of a precaution against dermal sensitization due to overexposure). If in doubt, highly dilute the mandarin in your blends, especially if you will be exposed to the sun. Store properly in the refrigerator, and do not use oxidized oils.

**Shelf life:** 1 to 2 years

## Sweet Orange

*Familiar—Welcoming—Tonic*

**Common names:** Sweet orange, orange

**Latin name:** *Citrus sinensis*

**Botanical family:** Rutaceae, primarily shrubs and trees and some herbs, commonly called the citrus family due to the high level of fruit-bearing citrus trees; also called the rue family. The family comprises 160 genera and more than 2,000 species; the majority grow in warm, temperate, or tropical regions.

**Attributes:** Orange is always smiling; there's always something wonderful in the world and it wants to share this feeling with you. Familiar, upbeat, cheerful, and happy, it is always having a good day and can help you have one, too.

**Character:** A medium-height tree, slightly taller than its cousin the mandarin, reaching up to 49 feet. In common with many of its citrus relatives, fragrant white blossoms appear before fruit is produced. In 1520, Portuguese travelers and explorers brought this botanical plant back from China after their expeditions, and so it was originally known as the "Portugal orange." Along with its cousin the lemon, traveled the ocean later to be grown in the New World. Medicinally, and as food, has been a symbol of good luck, dispelling congestion of the mind and body. Traditional Chinese Medicine, as well as more modern remedies, include orange for digestive and antianxiety issues. In Ayurveda, considered a nice tonic for reducing the heaviness and/or buzzing vibrations anxiety can bring. The vitamin C in

## Relax Personal Inhaler After Surgery
### (and digestive boost)

Add the following essential oils to a personal inhaler to aid in stimulating digestion before or after a meal—especially helpful when good nutrition can aid in recovery:

10 to 12 drops sweet orange

6 to 8 drops cardamom

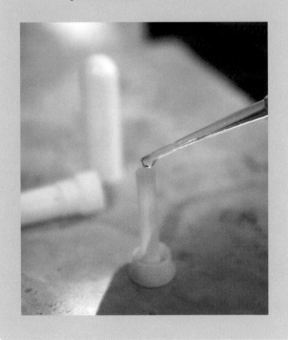

orange fruit has helped relieve scurvy (remember, essential oils contain no vitamins or minerals). As an essential oil, used as flavoring for the food and beverage industry, as well as its zest, which is what holds its concentrated oils.

**Unique aroma:** Citrusy, fresh, light, sweet, orange, clear, bright and warm

**Aromatic note:** Top

**Part of plant used for essential oils:** Peel, zest by expression (expressed sweet orange is considered nonphototoxic)

**Countries of origin:** Originally from Asia, now cultivated and distilled throughout Israel, Spain, Italy, and the United States, especially California and Florida.

**Special chemical properties:** Contains very high d-limonene (up to 95%).

**Actions:** Analgesic, antidepressant, antibacterial antifungal, antiseptic, antiviral, deodorant, digestive tonic, reduces anxiety, sedative, soothes nervous system, stimulant

**Uses:**

- *Physically:* Calms the mental and emotion components of stress-induced digestive upsets, which is beneficial to better body functioning. Relieves nausea, indigestion, flatulence, constipation, and even irritable bowels. Add to diffusers to relieve congestion in the airways and sinuses and to provide air purification. Also aids sore muscles and joints, gives skin and hair support with sebum-balancing, antiseptic, and anti-inflammatory actions for rashes, eczema, psoriasis, and insect bites.

- *Mentally:* In Traditional Chinese Medicine, calming the mind calms the *shen*, the vital essence considered the spiritual element of the human psyche. It is one of the "three treasures" of the human constitution, bridging the gap between the mind, body, emotional heart, and the spirit. Sweet orange is a wonderful tonic to calm the *shen*. With a calm mind, decisions are easier, focus is clearer, and the disposition is approachable and pleasant.

- *Emotionally:* Along with the previously discussed mental benefits, soothes anxiety, nervous tension, stress-induced fear and frustrations, depression, and SAD (seasonal affective disorder). Add to a diffuser in the wintertime or on cloudy days. During holidays, popularly diffused with spices, such as cardamom, cinnamon, or clove (all of which are oils with high dermal toxicity potential and need to be used with care outside of the diffuser), will awaken digestion and create an atmosphere of positivity and warmth. When the emotions turn outward to uncontrollable behaviors, such as compulsive or obsessive actions, this essential oil may be supportive.

- *Spiritually:* Optimism is a spiritual endeavor of the mind and emotional heart. This oil can brighten your spirit just as does sunshine the first thing every morning and uplifted lips in a satisfied smile at the end of the day.

**Blends well with:** Bergamot, black pepper, cardamom, cedarwood, clary sage, eucalyptus, fennel, frankincense, ginger, grapefruit, jasmine, laurel, lavender, lemon, mandarin, marjoram, neroli, oakmoss, palmarosa, palo santo, patchouli, peppermint, pine, Roman chamomile, rose geranium, rose, sandalwood, vanilla, vetiver, ylang-ylang

**Precautions:** Always dilute for topical application, to avoid skin irritation. Sweet orange is one of the few citrus oils considered to be nonphototoxic and one of the safer and gentlest essential oils for various ages; however, some sources suggest caution with *all* citrus essential oils applied to the skin, as a general safety guideline (which might be more of a precaution against dermal sensitization due to overexposure). If in doubt, highly dilute the orange in your blends, especially if you will be exposed to the sun. Store properly in the refrigerator, and do not use oxidized oils.

**Shelf life:** 1 to 2 years

# Juniper Berry
*Cleansing—Clearing—Focus*

**Common name:** Juniper berry

**Latin name:** *Juniperus communis*

**Botanical family:** Cupressaceae, also known as the cypress family, which includes cypress and redwood; one of the conifer families spanning the globe from forests to deserts. It is believed that this family first appeared during the Mesozoic Era (252.2 to 66 million years ago).

**Attributes:** Fruit of ancient wisdom, juniper is purifying, balancing, and may help you discern what you do not need and regain focus on what is in front of you.

**Character:** Not a tall tree, juniper is more stout and shrubby than long, sometimes growing to 6 feet tall, but can reach up to 25 feet high. There are more than 50 species of junipers, all sharing therapeutic values, all over the world; their scent may be different depending on their environment. Juniper's narrow evergreen leaves look flattened around its small bunches of berries. Used since antiquity, has been part of many important rituals, religious ceremonies, and purifications of air and body, and used as a preservative in ancient Egypt and Greece. In Britain, used to expel suspected unwanted energy from the house when burned in a fireplace and to protect the families from perceived witchcraft. Used by Egyptians and Native Americans for cleansing ceremonies and as incense in Tibetan ceremonies. In the 1800s, French hospitals burned the berries (which would release their essential oil) as a fumigant to prevent the spread of smallpox (Mojay 1997). This is the berry used to make gin.

**Unique aroma:** Piney, bittersweet, balsamic, woody, refreshing, slightly fruity, soft turpentine note.

**Aromatic note:** Base to mid

**Part of plant used for essential oils:** Berries

**Countries of origin:** Northern Europe, southwest Asia, North America

**Special chemical properties:** Primary constituents are the monoterpenes $\alpha$-pinene, $\beta$-pinene, and myrcene.

**Actions:** Analgesic, antiseptic, antiseborrheic, antiinflammatory, antifungal, antiviral, decongestant, detoxifier, increasing circulation, reducing fever

**Uses:**

- *Physically:* Can be used as a diuretic, antiseptic, and anti-inflammatory to cleanse the body, as a bath, local wash, in sitz baths (maximum dilution 2%), or in compresses. Use for steam inhalation to clear airways and sinuses and pores, cellulite, and even bronchitis. In times of stagnant, poor, or unmoving circulation, when muscles and joints are sore and stiff, can assist with cramping, rheumatic discomfort, and sprains and strains as well as stopped fluid, such as edema and swelling. Can act as a rubefacient, which helps bring fresh blood and oxygen to areas in need, and as a lymphatic mover to aid in eliminating waste from the body so it can run more efficiently. Relieves pain and has a slight drying action, so beneficial to skin that is slow to heal, reducing inflammation. Add to blends for astringent actions, such as for acne, sebum harmonization (especially if too oily) for skin and scalp, and eczema. Can be added to mouthwashes and antiviral blends, as for herpes. In Traditional Chinese Medicine, used to support the kidneys, spleen, and pancreas as a "kidney yang tonic"; used by Native Americans for colds, flu, and arthritic conditions.
- *Mentally:* As a stimulant of mind and body, can aid cloudy thoughts, confusion, low energy levels, and unmotivated stalls. Its warming actions can assist the body by hitting an invigorating Reset button in the mind.
- *Emotionally:* Just as a sluggish river can-

## Spot Treatment Sore Muscle/Joint Rub
### (adapted from David Crow's Joint Blend)

Create the following synergy in a ½-ounce amber or cobalt blue glass bottle:

8 drops juniper berry
4 drops *Eucalyptus globulus*
4 drops rosemary ct. verbenone
4 drops marjoram
2 drops ginger

Top the bottle off with a carrier blend of helichrysum herbal infused oil/jojoba blend (50/50 ratio). Close the cap and gently roll around to synergize all the oils and carriers together. Rub on sore joints and muscles as needed. (This is a 5% dilution to be used only for spot treatments, not full body application.)

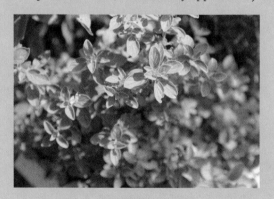

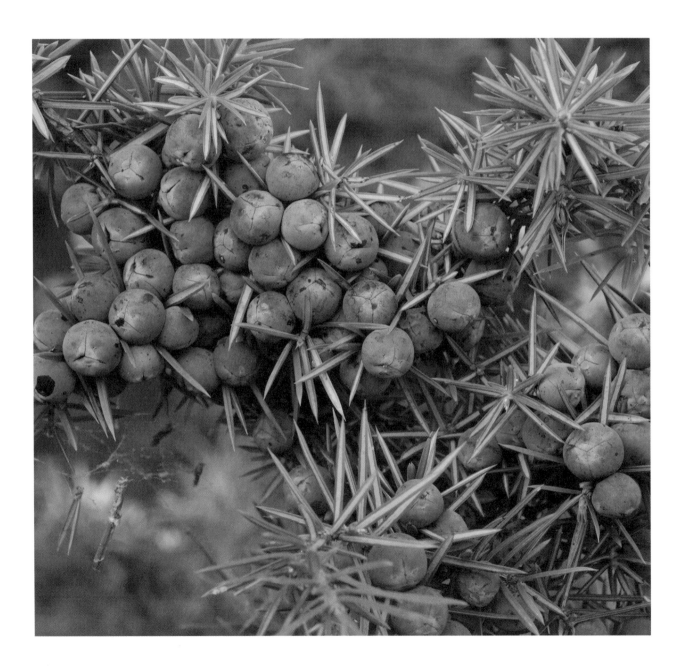

not move smoothly and ice is a solid block, emotions can slow you down or stop you all together. Use this essential oil when you lack the fluidity of ease in coping, or experience slow, paralyzing emotions, such as fear or worry, or feel blocked and completely stopped (frozen). Juniper's warming, ancient nature can teach adaptability, reaching out with a hand to bring you forward, one step at a time, so you are no longer standing in one spot. Juniper has survived many moons and can show you there is a way to see the sun.

- *Spiritually:* Ancient wisdom can be found in the old trees. The essential oils from juniper and woods and resins (see Chapter 12) are innately and deeply connected to the time-honored ways of nature and humanity. Perseverance is one of them. Juniper's small berries hold the potential to help in times of transition, moving from stagnation of the spirit toward lighter spiritual freedom.

**Blends well with:** Cedarwood, clary sage, cypress, *Eucalyptus globulus* or *E. radiata*, fennel, frankincense, geranium, grapefruit, helichrysum, lavender, lemon, mandarin, palo santo, pine, rosemary ct. verbenone, sandalwood, sweet orange, vetiver

**Precautions:** Store in the refrigerator; do not use old or oxidized oils. Skin sensitivity is high if oxidized oil is used. For topical applications, it is suggested to add an antioxidant to the blend.

**Shelf life:** 2 to 3 years

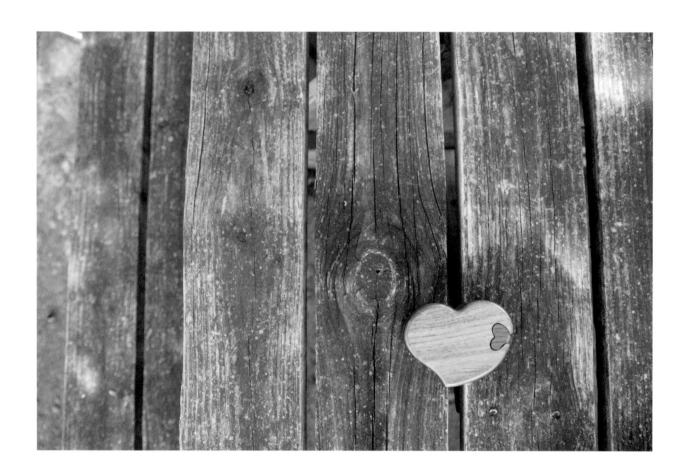

# CHAPTER 12

# Woods and Resins

*There is a pleasure in the pathless woods, / There is a rapture in the lonely shore, / There is society where none intrudes, / By the deep Sea, and music in its roar: / I love not Man the less, but Nature more . . .* —Lord Byron, *Childe Harold*

## Fortitude—Stability— Deep Healing

Woods signify stability, anchored motion, support, longevity and wisdom, slowing down. Their resins represent self-healing, healing the inner wounds of experience, bringing inspiration forward from the unseen, seeing within, protection, unwavering strength but flexibility.

Trees provide comfortable passage beneath their canopies of shade, purify the air, and bring the world a harmony of birdsong on their branches and wind through their leaves. Whether hundreds of feet tall or close to the earth, all tap into the powers of the sun, moon, earth, and rain. The Tree of Life has many interpretations but each concerns the imparting of wisdom from nature to mankind; an exchange of symbiotic honoring and respect.

*Important note:* Each of the following oils have the potential of being endangered due to over-harvesting. Honor these trees by using mindfully; purchase only what you need and what you will use. You will note an additional "precious oil" reminder in the oil profiles.

## Cedarwood

*Steady—Clearing—Reassuring*

**Precious oil:** Cedarwood is listed as possibly endangered; use mindfully, purchase with care.

**Common names:** Cedarwood, also known as Atlas cedar

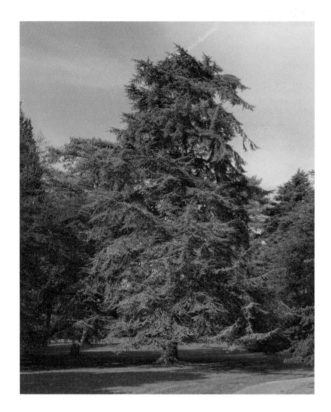

**Latin name:** *Cedrus atlantica*

**Botanical family:** Pinaceae, known for the great trees, such as pines, spruces, firs, hemlocks, and larches. Only Atlas cedar and the Himalayan cedars (*Cedrus deodora*) are in the Pinaceae family. Other cedars, such as Mexican cedar and Virginian cedar, belong to the Cupressaceae family.

**Attributes:** Steady, confident cedar is a strong, long-lasting wood and produces essential oils with respiratory, skin, fluid, and spiritual guidance.

**Character:** Cedar has long been valued for its abil-ity to resist fungus, insects, and decay; historically used for masts of ships, temples, palaces, doorways, and furniture throughout the Middle East. It is said to have been used for the Temple of Solomon, the first temple built in Jerusalem. Food preservation and the Egyptian mummification process included cedar. Most historically documented uses are believed to connect to the famed Lebanon cedars, which, after 3,000 years of heavy use, had been at risk of extinction until their current protection in a few small groves, known as the "Forest of the Cedars of Gods"; some of which trees are estimated to be 2,500 years old. Atlas cedar is a descendant of Lebanon cedars, and while it does not reach their height (up to 165 feet), it can grow as high as 40 to 60 feet, and even occasionally to 130 feet. As does sandalwood, cedar builds its essential oils within its wood over time; the older the tree base, the more oil it produces. Harvesting old trees can mean the increased need for reforestation to maintain the longevity of the species. It takes a generation to produce cedar's essential oils.

**Unique aroma:** Warm, woody, sweet, balsamic, slightly camphoraceous, slightly smoky, subtle hint of spice. While some consider cedar to be masculine, it appeals to both sexes due to its soft woody scent.

**Aromatic note:** Mid to base

**Part of plant used for essential oils:** Wood, steam distilled

**Countries of origin:** Morocco in particular, and the Atlas Mountains of Algeria, but cedar's ancestors and cousins are deeply connected to the Mediterranean area, as well as the Taiga biome.

## Subtle and Gentle: Uplift, Be Steady, Be Clear

Add to a water room diffuser:

2 drops cedarwood

2 drops eucalyptus

2 drops sweet orange

For children over age 2, only diffuse for 10 to 15 minutes, then turn off. Substitute rosalina for eucalyptus or eliminate eucalyptus for younger children.

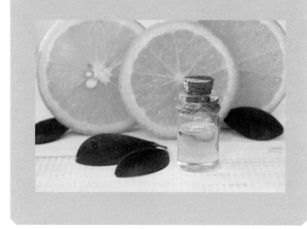

**Actions:** Antifungal, antiseptic, astringent, breaks up mucus, calmative, insect repellent, lymphatic decongestant, general tonic

**Uses:**

- *Physically:* Best known for its ability to fight off infections in the lungs and airways. Add to blends when there is congestion, viral, fungal, and/or bacterial issues, including colds, flu, and coughs. When mucus is a problem, try using with a bit of eucalyptus or your choice of pine or fir in a diffuser, steam inhalation, or chest rub. Considered to be purifying and cleansing. Its astringent nature may be helpful in blends that aid eczema that is moist, acne, excess sebum on the face or scalp, concerns of hair loss, and dandruff. Insect-repelling; a good match for skin infections concerning lice, scabies, or worms. Use when the circulation system needs a boost, or for aches and pains in the muscles or joints. Can be used with children.

- *Mentally:* Considered a stabilizing essential oil. Its warm and dry nature may help you find steadiness in your decisions. Encourages mental energy and focus in a calm, steady pace when things are feeling unproductive, without causing a need for fast-paced immediate action.

- *Emotionally:* When irritability, anxiety, or fear swirl from different directions, can help locate the calmness in the storm. Can assist with finding the place that feels most appropriate to you, rather than what the outside influences are pressuring you to do; to hold you steady and secure in what feels right to you, and help you find your sense of will.

- *Spiritually:* Use in your meditations when there is need to connect to the ancient wisdom of the planet and your own divine source. Cedar is not a source of words, but a deeper place of being.

**Blends well with:** Bergamot, cistus, cypress, grapefruit, jasmine, juniper berry, lavender, lemon, mandarin, neroli, patchouli, rose geranium, rose, rosemary, sweet orange, ylang-ylang

**Precautions:** Do not use old or oxidized oils. Store in the refrigerator.

**Shelf life:** 6 to 8+ years

# Frankincense

*Ancient—Wisdom—Inner Healing*

**Precious oil:** Use frankincense mindfully, as it is listed as potentially endangered. Husbandry of the trees has diminished due to political and cultural changes.

**Common name:** Frankincense, from the Anglo-French *franc encens* ("high" and "incense")

**Latin names:** There are 25 frankincense species in the *Boswellia* genus, plus several synonyms. A few commonly used in aromatherapy: *Boswellia carteri*, a.k.a. *Boswellia carterii* (with two *i*'s); *Boswellia sacra*; *Boswellia frereana*; *Boswellia serrata*; *Boswellia papyrifera*.

**Botanical family:** Burseraceae, native to tropical environments; all are resinous trees and shrubs (all parts are aromatic, not just the resin!). Many are uniquely adapted to the desert, surviving long periods without rain. Frankincense's cousins are palo santo and myrrh.

**Attributes:** Soothing, grounding, stabilizing, inner healing, spiritual. Just as its bark, wood, flowers,

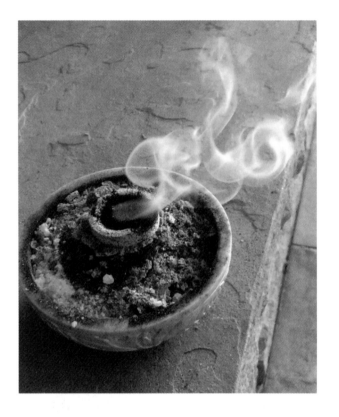

and fruit all share its scent, frankincense will help who you are inside resonate throughout your whole being and the overspill of greatness will touch others.

**Character:** Reaching heights of only 25 feet, frankincense is a shrubby tree, perfectly adapted to the desert terrain of North Africa and the Middle East. Its resin droplets, called tears, are collected around the tree, then slowly cured or hardened. They are then graded according to their translucency, their color—light yellow to dark brown—as well as from which country they came. The resin's history is long, its ancestry deeply steeped in relationship with the earth and her people. Once valued more than gold, frankincense was one of the gifts from the Magi in the biblical birth story of Jesus. Its first recorded use as a cosmetic was in Egyptian kohl (Isaac 2004). It has traveled the Silk Road. As an incense, has been in every human ritual, including births, deaths (such as embalming), and marriages, and has been one of the main ingredients in Sabbath ceremonial offerings in Judaism. One of the essential oils David Crow refers to as a "wish fulfilling gem" and a "sacred scent," indicating the legacy of its use in important spiritual connections, rituals, ceremonies, meditations, and prayers (2016).

**Unique aroma:** Fresh, earthy, woody, clean, citrusy, piney, rosy, floral, balsamic, slightly spicy, warm, resinous, rich, camphoraceous. *B. carteri* has the traditional frankincense scent, resinous, deeper, soft floral, and piney; *B. frereana* is lighter, pungent, balsamic; *B. papyrifera* is more floral, with softer citrus notes; *B. serrata* has higher citrusy notes with piney notes.

**Aromatic note:** Mid to midbase

**Part of plant used for essential oils:** Resin

**Countries of origin:** North Africa and the Middle East, specifically Oman and Somalia for distillation, as well as Ethiopia, Yemen, and China

**Special chemical properties:** Its high levels of the monoterpenes α-pinene and d-limonene (*B. carteri*) are particularly good for uplifting the mind and spirit.

## Facial Oil Skin Support
### (for acne or aging)

In a ½-ounce bottle, create the following synergy:

1 drop frankincense
1 drop rose geranium
1 drop patchouli
1 drop clary sage
1 drop helichrysum

Then, add a 1:1:1 mixture of almond oil, apricot kernel oil, and rosehip seed oil to the bottle. Cap with an orifice reducer, seal with the lid, and gently roll around to mix. Label properly. Use 2 to 3 drops morning and night. Tap oil on your face gently with fingertips after cleansing. Best stored in the refrigerator if rosehip seed is used.

**Actions:** Analgesic, antibacterial, antidepressant, anti-infectious, antimicrobial, astringent, immunity tonic, reduces anxiety, sedative, soothes nervous system, wound healing

**Uses:**

- *Physically:* While *Boswellia*'s different species may have some slightly different benefits depending on chemical constitution, all have similar immunity-boosting benefits. Add to a

such as hives. Include in rubs, gels, or salves to relieve muscular aches and pains, arthritis, carpel tunnel syndrome, rheumatism, and neuralgias.

- *Mentally:* Can lift the heaviness of emotions, which helps the mind think clearer while allowing it to be still.
- *Emotionally:* A relaxed emotional heart is a place of gentleness and ease—sleep comes and insomnia is abated. Frankincense helps you rise above the feeling of adversity, allowing you to connect to your inner strength and confidence, providing safe passage to your own ancient wisdom.
- *Spiritually:* Its resin symbolizes rising above perceived hardships or an unstable base, and that a life that is powerful does not need perfect conditions to be valued, respected, influential, and important. Add to meditative, contemplative, and/or spiritual practices.

**Blends well with:** Bergamot, cardamom, cistus, clary sage, fennel, frankincense species, grapefruit, jasmine, laurel, lavender, lemon, mandarin, neroli, patchouli, rose geranium, rose, rosemary, ylang-ylang

**Precautions:** Store in the refrigerator, as can oxidize with air and light exposure.

**Shelf life:** 1 to 3 years

## Palo Santo
*Centering—Meditative—Sacred*

**Precious oil:** Due to the time needed to obtain oil (a

blend to clear congestion in airways and provide lymph support. Assists with antiaging, wrinkles, scar and wound healing, acne, and inflamed or dry, irritated skin, such as eczema. Add to a synergy when pores are blocked (e.g., with blackheads) or to soothe inflammatory responses,

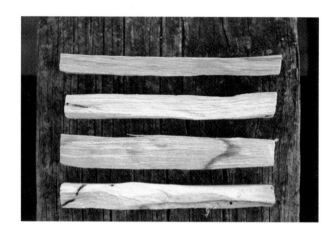

generation or more), use this oil with care, only purchasing what you will be using.

**Common name:** Palo santo, meaning "holy stick" or "holy wood" (originally called "sweet stick")

**Latin name:** *Bursera graveolens*. *Graveolens* is Latin for "heavy, penetrating odor."

**Botanical family:** Burseraceae, the same family as frankincense and myrrh (both potentially endangered gum resins), all of which are resinous trees and shrubs. Many plants in this family are uniquely adapted to the desert, surviving long periods without rain.

**Attributes:** Protective; spiritually and emotionally uplifting; self-regulating. Palo santo is sentient.

**Character:** A tree that grows as tall as 60 feet, with many branches, palo santo has been considered quite sacred and powerful by Incan shamans and indigenous peoples of Peru, Ecuador, Bolivia, and Brazil for hundreds if not thousands of years. The smoke from its burning wood is said to lighten the mind, uplift the heart, and repel insects. Its essential oils are obtained in ways unlike any others. The tree must live a natural life, approximately 50 years or longer (average life span is 80 to 90 years, but there are reports of much older trees), die a natural death, not by illness or disease, and it must not be cut down prematurely. After the death of the tree, it must be allowed to decompose naturally, on its own timeline, for at least three years, preferably six, before its essential oil may be obtained from the wood. "Female" trees share richer oil than "male" trees in both aroma and color. Intimately connected to the lunar cycle, from its death to the collection of its essential oils—the tree produces less at a new moon and more at a full moon—it grows in locations at the equator where it receives consistent sunlight each day of the year, except during the rainy season, when it uses the water to grow quickly (Crow 2012). It is now protected in Ecuador, where no living branches or trees are allowed to be cut. Dante Bolcato, a distiller of palo santo in Ecuador, believes the tree is cognizant of the people that connect to its essence, as well as the earth and the time it spends in nature (Crow 2012).

**Unique aroma:** Sweet, citrusy, fresh, resinous, woody, hidden powdery scent

**Aromatic note:** Top to mid

**Part of plant used for essential oils:** Naturally aged, dead wood from fallen trees

**Country of origin:** Ecuador

**Special chemical properties:** Palo santo's high d-limonene content (almost 65%) accounts for its sci-

> ## Meditation Blend
>
> Create the following synergy, then add to a base of apricot kernel carrier oil in a ½-ounce bottle. Use a drop on temples, wrists, and nape of the neck for morning meditations, before going to bed, or in meditative practices.
>
> 2 to 3 drops palo santo
>
> 2 to 3 drops frankincense
>
> 2 to 3 drops ginger (optional) for warming; *or* 2 to 3 drops rose geranium (optional) for self-love; *or* 2 to 3 drops lavender (optional) for resting, evening

entifically proven antidepressant qualities used by shamans and their ancestors for generations via the resin in the wood as it burned. A single drop of the oil can be placed within the palms, rubbed vigorously, then inhaled as a palm inhalation, or placed in a personal inhaler, for relaxing properties, to open creativity, and ease emotional and respiratory distress.

**Actions:** Antidepressant, antiseptic, anti-inflammatory, immunity supportive, antimicrobial, insect repellent, sedative, reduces anxiety

**Uses:**

- *Physically:* Harmonizes sebum production, especially in acne or oily skin; also good in skin-care blends for antiaging and antioxidant purposes. Use for muscular and joint aches and pains as well as rheumatism, and neuralgias. Add to a synergy for respiratory issues, such as infections, coughs, congestion, asthma and allergies, colds, and flu (works well in chest rubs for people of all ages).

- *Mentally:* A unique oil, reiterating that the mental, emotional, and spiritual aspects of any person are not separate, but one. In Ayurveda, used to pacify any of the doshas that are exhibiting excess attributes. In Traditional Chinese Medicine, promotes the flow of qi.

- *Emotionally:* Known throughout the ages by indigenous peoples and wise men for its antidepressant support, calming the emotions of sadness, anxiety, panic attacks, nervousness, and distress. Palo santo symbolizes the return to center, the place where the earth and sky meet, the fire of sun at the equator of the planet, cooled by the moon's waning and waxing. It knows the aridness of desert and the fulfilment of a torrential rainstorm. By surviving extremes, it understands centering.

- *Spiritually:* Palo santo is restorative. It has been used in religious and spiritual ceremonies, incense burning, and in fire altars for many suns and moons as a sacred wood. Its resinous essential oil has been said to connect to the greater spiritual forces with a divine intelligence. Valuable in meditative and contemplative spaces, it supports the inner nature and creativity. David Crow identifies palo santo as one of the "wish fulfilling gems" and sacred scents that include frankincense, myrrh, and sandalwood. Connecting with palo santo also teaches how to regulate the notion of giving and taking. It teaches boundaries, to not be taken advantage of, as well as to know when to give with abundance. Gratitude and deep honor are among its attributes.

**Blends well with:** Cedarwood, clary sage, cypress, fir, fragonia, frankincense, ginger, grapefruit, jasmine, lavender, lemon, mandarin, neroli, palmarosa, patchouli, rose geranium, rose, sandalwood, spruce, sweet orange, valerian, vetiver, ylang-ylang

**Precautions:** There are no known precautions associated with palo santo, except to store in the refrigerator and to avoid skin sensitization by avoiding and discarding oxidized essential oils.

**Shelf life:** 1 to 2 years

# Sandalwood

*Heart-centered—Harmonizer—Ancient*

**Precious oil:** *S. album*, the most widely known sandalwood oil is an endangered species. Australian sandalwood, *S. spicatum*, is sustainable and will most likely be changing the world of sandalwood use. Purchase *S. album* with care

**Common name:** Sandalwood

**Latin name:** *Santanlum album*

**Botanical family:** Santalaceae, a group of herbs, shrubs, and trees happy in dry areas of tropical and temperate environments with semiparasitic requirements for survival. Relying on the host plant to pro-

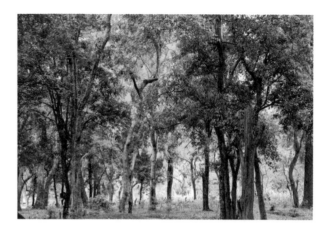

vide minerals and nutrients, this family is especially connected to the roots of the host plants.

**Attributes:** Connects to the heart, the deep center, the equilibrium, and the pulse of living. Calming, centering, enticing.

**Character:** Sandalwood is in danger of being overharvested; it is important to choose oil only from sustainable, ethical resources dedicated to reforestation. Like cedarwood, sandalwood must be allowed to reach maturity to produce valuable essential oils. They are symbols of time, perseverance, and care. It takes sandalwood 30 to 50 years to reach maturity, depending on growing conditions. It can reach heights just under 30 feet and produces small purple flowers. The only place *aromatic* essential oils are located in its entire botanical makeup is within the heartwood. All other oils within its branches and roots are odorless. No other essential oil has a scent quite like sandalwood. It is one of the oldest known perfumes recorded.

## Peaceful Night Anointing Oil Blend

Add to a ½-ounce bottle of your choice of carrier (almond, coconut, apricot kernel):

1 to 3 drops sandalwood
1 to 3 drops lavender
1 to 2 drops sweet orange or neroli

Blend together in a gentle rolling action. When applying this oil to wrists, behind the ears, sternum, or crown of the head, hold in your heart the intention of calmness, an open heart, and a connection to the pulse of our innermost wisdom. Take a moment to simply be with the blend. Can be applied to enjoy your day or to rest well at night.

Ayurveda has a wonderful word: *sāttvik* (*SAHT-vik*). A person, place, thing, food, or environment can be *sāttvik*. It is the essence of true being, without disturbance, containing mental and emotional peacefulness, without waves to complicate things. For example, when eating, one must strive to eat a *sāttvik* meal in a *sāttvik* environment, meaning a meal with foods that work with your body, not against it, and in an environment that is peaceful. When using essential oils, the goal is always to create a *sāttvik* experience. Sandalwood and many of the other woods and resins have an innate *sāttvik* capability. The magic of this kind of peacefulness is it is not always immediately obvious, but subtle and gentle.

Highly valued in traditional and cultural practices throughout Asia and India, in Buddhist and Hindu rituals, and as incense and in scented wooded carvings, furniture, and temple structures. Ayurveda and Traditional Chinese Medicine have long used sandalwood for the ability to soothe and calm the body, mind, and spirit.

**Unique aroma:** Soft, woody, smooth, rich, earthy, nutty, sweet, balsamic, slightly musky, a whisper of powdery scent

**Aromatic note:** Base
**Part of plant used for essential oils:** Wood, heart-wood of the trunk, and/or sawdust
**Countries of origin:** India, Indonesia, and several Asian regions. There are different species in Australia and in the Hawaiian Islands.
**Special chemical properties:** Its highest components are cis-$\alpha$(alpha)-santalol, cis-$\beta$(beta)-santalol, and cis-laceol, all sesquiterpene alcohols.
**Actions:** Antibacterial, antidepressant, anti-inflammatory, antimicrobial, antiviral, aphrodisiac, sedative, soothes nervous system, general tonic
**Uses:**

- *Physically:* Used to quell "hot" conditions of inflammation of mucous membranes, digestion, and skin. Soothes bug bites, acne, and even cold sores. Harmonizes sebum production, especially when the skin is dry or chapped. Use in blends for mature skin and for irritations from razor burn or abrasions. Adding to an abdominal massage may assist with flatulence, bloating, and digestive upsets. Add to blends to assist with dry or hot throats, laryngitis, dry irritated nasal passageways, dry coughs, and bronchitis. May relieve urinary tract concerns by adding to a sitz bath along with juniper berry. (Always consult a doctor to find the source of the problem.)

- *Mentally:* Famously used to bridge the well-being of body, mind, and spirit together through the heart. The calm, sedative actions of this aroma are pleasing to the mind, supporting the center, especially when feeling overwhelmed.
- *Emotionally:* Use to disperse hot emotions, such as anger, frustration, and irritation, which upset the equilibrium of the body. Relieves disturbed sleep, headaches, and nervous agitation. Aids the centering of emotions, such as anxiety, soothing and opening the emotional heart.
- *Spiritually:* One of the longest recorded scents for spiritual and aromatic ceremonial and ritual. Said to promote inner awareness, heightened consciousness, creativity, and peace of mind; to mute the distractions of nonbeneficial thought; and to reveal beneficial spiritual endeavors.

**Blends well with:** Bergamot, cedarwood, frankincense, jasmine, lavender, mandarin, neroli, palo santo, patchouli, rose geranium, rose, sweet orange, vetiver, ylang-ylang

**Precautions:** True sandalwood in its pure form does not have any skin-irritating factors in proper dilution; however, sandalwood is commonly adulterated with chemicals that can raise dermal sensitivity. Proper dilution ratios always advised.

**Shelf life:** 4 to 8+ years. (Mark Webb reports he has sandalwood that is over 20 years old; with proper storage, it can be maintained a long time, the same as patchouli!)

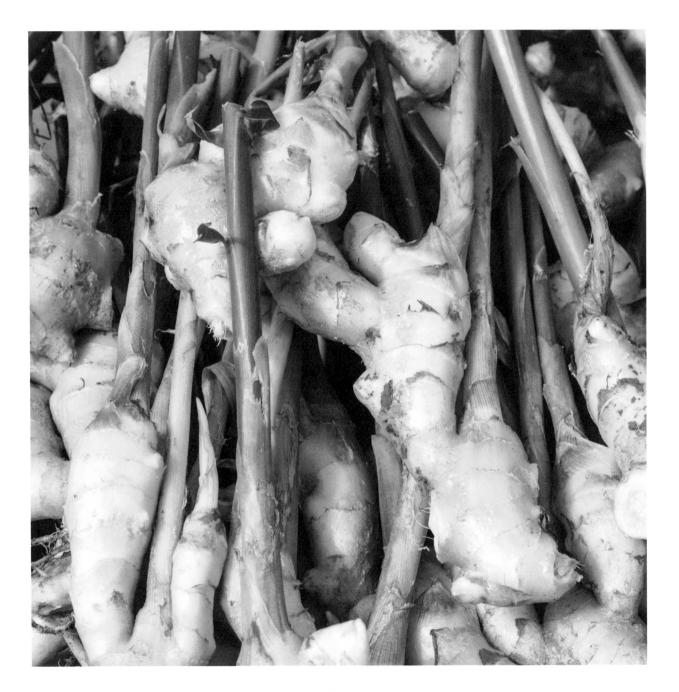

# CHAPTER 13

# Roots and Rhizomes

*Deep in their roots, all flowers keep the light.* —Theodore Roethke

## Grounded—Nurtured—Mystery

Roots and rhizomes hold groundedness, deep resources, warmth, encouragement. While providing connection to the sun and moon, the wind and rain, they symbolize the safety and feeling of coming home, its stability and comfort. Roots are steadfast, the source behind the visible. The root of a plant gathers its nutrients and quenches its thirst by soaking up water. Rhizomes, with their ability to grow laterally, embody the idea of family, each node creating an offshoot to start another plant, the connection to the deeper self. There is a bit of a mystery to roots and rhizomes, for not everyone remembers them beneath the ground, a hidden world below the visible foliage. But they are where secret communications are coded in through beneficial bacteria and fungus, connecting the plant to the soil in even more layers and finer levels of contact.

## Ginger

*Warming—Encouraging—Stimulating*
**Common name:** Ginger
**Latin name:** *Zingiber officinalis*
**Botanical family:** Zingiberaceae, also known as the ginger family; includes other herbs and spices, such as turmeric, used for culinary and medicinal pur-

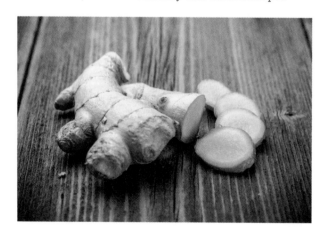

poses. Heavily tropical, with many ornamental and flowering varieties.

**Attributes:** Warming, grounding, and stimulating; promotes long life and strength.

**Character:** Any time you see *officinalis* in a Latin binomial, you know there are many uses pertaining to medicinal value within the plant. Ginger has been recognized for such value for thousands of years. It can grow as high as 3 feet, with stalks that go upward, decorated with narrow leafy foliage and blooms of white, yellow, or purple resembling the delicate orchid's design. Although often called a root, it is a rhizome, a knobby cork-colored structure with the ability to reproduce from the nodes branched off from the main piece—it can be cut into pieces and a new plant propagated. Ginger spreads linearly, rather than downward like a root. It likes heat and tropical areas, especially in India, China, and other Asian regions. For thousands of years, it has been used by Romans, Greeks, Arabs, Chinese, and the Spanish. It crossed the Atlantic to the West Indies. Now, it is grown in warm, moist botanical gardens and backyards for culinary and decorative purposes. Its historic medicinal uses include warming the body to sweat out illness (increasing circulation) as well as a digestive stimulant and nausea reliever.

**Unique aroma:** Warm, spicy, pungent, sweet, woody, sharp, whisper of earthiness

**Aromatic note:** Mid to base

**Part of plant used for essential oils:** Rhizome (preferably unpeeled)

**Countries of origin:** Tropical India and Southeast Asia

**Special chemical properties:** Has a unique chemical component called α-zingiberene, one of a few chemicals that gives it its distinctive aroma and acts as an anti-inflammatory.

**Actions:** Analgesic, antibacterial, antispasmodic, digestive support, immunity harmonizer, rubefacient

**Uses:**

- *Physically:* Famous for its warming digestive tonic properties. Relieves stomach upsets, especially flatulence, gas, and bloating with a clockwise abdominal massage. Can reduce nausea, which pregnant women (inhalation) and those with travel sickness may appreciate (try in a personal inhaler with sweet orange). Helpful in blends to allay cold: cold feet, cold hands, as well as for colds and flu. Bronchial concerns with "cold" phlegm can be aided by adding to a personal inhaler, diffuser, or chest rubs along with eucalyptus (age 6 and older) and pine. Add to diffusers during times of seasonal change, when respiratory and allergy-related indicators tend to appear. Add to blends for muscle aches and pains and for athletes who want to "warm up" their muscles and joints on a cold day. Beneficial for pain associated with stiffness and coldness, such as rheumatic pain. For peripheral warmth, try adding a drop of black pepper and one of the analgesic pines or juniper berry. For menstrual

## Digestive Stimulant

To encourage digestion at a meal and to assist with appetite, add the following to a room diffuser, running for 20 minutes before the meal and/or during the meal:

1 drop ginger
1 drop fennel
1 drop cardamom
1 drop black pepper

If pregnant or nursing simply inhale ginger from a personal inhaler.

discomfort, try with cardamom, clary sage, or Roman chamomile. Can be used in aphrodisiac blends, especially for frigidity and impotence (try with sandalwood, patchouli, and jasmine or ylang-ylang).

- *Mentally:* Warms the mind to thoughts of action; removes slow, unmotivated frozen blocks; ignites confidence and the charisma of positivity. Use to ignite focus with soft warmth.
- *Emotionally:* Provides warmth throughout the nervous system to calm anxious or nervous emotions, especially if associated with overwhelming exhaustion. When you lack the energy to "dig deeper," picture how, as a rhizome, ginger feels supported by the earth all around where its growth yet continues, allowed to happen naturally. This is empowering, comforting, and strengthening, particularly when depletion and fatigue has been lingering. If you find you tend to "pick up" other people's energy and emotions, grounding essential oils, such as ginger and vetiver can be helpful in stabilizing your center.
- *Spiritually:* Ginger's warming scent is unique, as are you. There is no one like you. Ginger can help you "root" into your source of being, adding stimulating and encouraging aromatic benefits to meditations, quiet moments, and when action is needed. Add to room diffusers holding the space for affection and passion.

**Blends well with:** Black pepper, cardamom, cedarwood, clary sage, cypress, frankincense, grapefruit, helichrysum, jasmine, laurel, lavender, lemon, lemongrass, marjoram, neroli, palo santo, patchouli, rose geranium, sandalwood, sweet fennel, sweet orange, vetiver

**Precautions:** Ginger is generally nonirritating, has GRAS status, and is highly utilized in both Ayurveda and Traditional Chinese Medicine. However, its essential oil is quite warming topically and should be diluted to 1% or less if going to be applied to the skin in any way (carrier, bath, compress) (Crow 2016). It takes very little to make a big impact with this essential oil. Start with a low number of drops. You can always add more, but you cannot take away. If you are pregnant, using ginger in an inhaler may help reduce nausea, but be sure to ask your doctor first and consult with a qualified aromatherapist for safe use.

**Shelf life:** 4 to 5 years

# Vetiver

*Grounding—Connecting—Restorative*

**Common names:** Vetiver, also known as khus-khus

**Latin name:** *Vetiveria zizanoides*

**Botanical family:** Poaceae, also called Graminaea, the grass family, home to genera of grass, rice, bamboo, sugar, and reeds. You may recognize vetiver's aromatic cousins lemongrass, citronella, and palmarosa. They grow all over the globe in various terrains.

**Attributes:** Nourishes the spirit by supporting the body; grounding. Known as the "oil of tranquility" in Sri Lanka.

**Character:** Grows in clumps with thick bundles of roots that branch off a rhizome structure. The root system does not go deep; however, it is abundant. The roots change from white to yellow in maturity, contrasting the new and the established. Vetiver yields very little oil, making it costly to produce. The essential oil is quite thick and viscous, influenced heavily by the color of the earth, golden brown to dark brown. It has been historically used in perfumes as a fixative, inviting other more volatile essential oils to stay awhile longer, rather than disperse too quickly. Traditionally, has been used to scent ward-

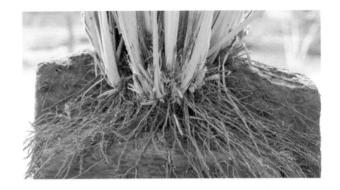

robes and rooms; its grass blades have been woven into mats and screens to ward off insects. One of the few oils that improves with age (like patchouli).

**Unique aroma:** Deep, earthy, warm, woody, sweet, rich, resinous, slightly smoky

**Aromatic note:** Deep base

**Part of plant used for essential oils:** Root

**Countries of origin:** Haiti, Sri Lanka, and India, Réunion islands

**Actions:** Antiseptic, antispasmodic, anti-inflammatory, digestive stimulant, immunity booster, sedative, skin support, soothes nervous system

**Uses:**

- *Physically:* The soft, comforting sedative action of this essential oil can promote sleep, revitalization, and rejuvenation. Repels insects. Use for acne, wounds and abrasions, stretch marks, and to harmonize oily skin and eczema. Reduces inflammation of muscles, joints, stiffness, arthritis, and rheumatism. Helpful when the immune system appears to be stalled, fatigued, or low. Provides support for varicose veins, cold hands or feet, and poor circulation as well in times of excess heat. Has an innately nourishing nature and it may counteract malabsorption of nutrients, weight loss, loss of appetite, and anemia (Mojay 1997). Note: Only a doctor can diagnose anemia, and if you have anemia, you should get your doctor's permission before you use vetiver.

- *Mentally:* Has been used in traditional practices of Ayurveda for mood and concentration and in Traditional Chinese Medicine to calm and nourish the mind and body (Crow 2016). Calms the overheated mind (Mojay 1997).
- *Emotionally:* In Ayurveda, has been used for nervousness, exhaustion, eating disorders, stress, and to enhance romantic moods (Crow 2016). Can boost confidence, without a push for action, but by cooling and settling into a sense of security. Use for "flightiness" or feeling disconnected from the physicality of your body. Add a rose-scented oil (such as rose, rose geranium, or palmarosa) or jasmine to enhance the feeling of beauty, self-love, and heart-centeredness.
- *Spiritually:* Especially helpful if spiritual spaces and/or meditations result in spaciness, or for those who often "travel upward" in their quiet spaces or have feelings of being out of their body. Embodies the connection to your mental, emotional, and physical being, allowing you to be rooted, grounded, and connected to your experience here in this moment. At the same time, many may find vetiver to be uplifting, like the scent after a rain.

**Blends well with:** Bergamot, black pepper, cardamom, cedarwood, clary sage, cypress, fir, frankincense, ginger, grapefruit, helichrysum, jasmine, laurel, lavender, lemongrass, marjoram, neroli, palmarosa, palo santo, patchouli, pine, rose geranium, rose, sandalwood, sweet orange, ylang-ylang

**Precautions:** Generally nonirritating, but be mindful: this oil may contain isoeugenol, to which some people are allergic (Shutes 2015). Also, vetiver is incredibly persistent and penetrating; one drop can last for days, so make sure you mean to use it. Very viscous (thick), so using in a room diffuser may prove problematic (instead, try one drop on a cotton ball and you'll smell it in the whole room with no problem). Use in a personal inhaler for a more individual experience.

**Shelf life:** 4 to 8+ years

---

## Grounding and Calming Blend

Create a personal inhaler with the following essential oils (this blend is too thick for a diffuser):

3 drops vetiver

3 drops rose or rose geranium or palmarosa

2 drops jasmine

2 drops patchouli

4 drops mandarin or sweet orange

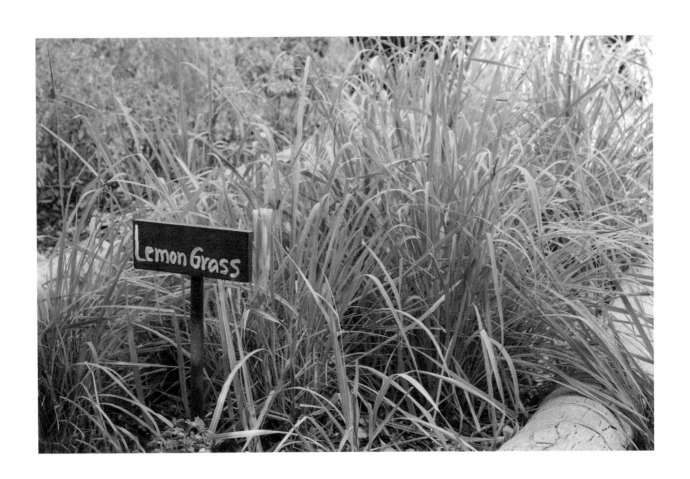

# CHAPTER 14

# Grasses

*I believe the leaf of grass is no less than the journey-work of the stars.*
—Walt Whitman, *Song of Myself*

## Flexible—Dispelling—Freedom

Grasses represent the ability to remain anchored with flexibility, movement, and grounded lightness, the freedom to see more than one side of an issue, and group support.

Each individual blade must adapt to the environmental changes from the sun, moon, soil, rain, and wind. The connection to the earth is quite intimate as grasses are adaptive to the growing conditions of the terrain. Only certain grasses grow in certain soils, some suited quite well to what would otherwise be a challenging environment. There is safety in knowing they have freedom yet will not fly away. Grasses around the world have been used medicinally, decoratively, and to protect the land from erosion.

## Lemongrass
*Uplifting—Cleansing—Stimulating*

**Common name:** Lemongrass
**Latin name:** *Cymbopogon citratus*
**Botanical family:** Poaceae, also called Graminaea, known as the grass family, also home to vetiver and palmarosa. Its genera comprise grass, rice, bamboo, sugar, and reeds, which grow all over the globe in various terrains, and produce 50 to 60 aromatic grasses.
**Attributes:** Especially useful for circulation, toning, revitalizing, digestive, and antifungal purposes. Lemongrass supplies warm movement and dispels windy/cold ailments of the mind and body.
**Character:** Can grow up to 3 feet tall with long, sharp-edged blades of lemon-scented grass. Although distilled for its essential oils, this botan-

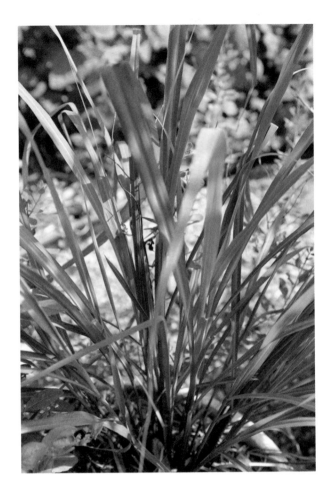

goods, such as perfume, cleaning products, food, pharmaceuticals, and tobacco (Shutes 2016).

**Unique aroma:** Lemony, fresh, uplifting, strong, penetrating

**Aromatic note:** Top to mid

**Part of plant used for essential oils:** Grass

**Countries of origin:** Native to tropical regions of Southeast Asia, but can be found in Nepal, the West Indies, and South Africa

**Actions:** Analgesic, antidepressant, antiviral, immunity booster, general tonic

**Uses:**

- *Physically:* Its antifungal, antibacterial, and antiviral activities help purify the air after an illness (in a diffuser and used for cleaning). These same properties relieve athlete's foot, ringworm, and candida. Include in your atmosphere and skin preparations for rashes, eczema, psoriasis, and when skin is the indicator of internal stress. Brightens skin tone, harmonizes sebum production, and has antioxidant properties useful for

ical plant has been used for thousands of years in indigenous medicinal preparations as a tea. The grass itself is used in Asian cuisine to give a lemony flavor. Lemongrass's historic connection to food and medicine is extensive throughout South and Southeast Asia as well as in Guatemala and Brazil. It has also been used to scent and flavor commercial topical applications. Where there is sluggishness, such as cellulite, and sagging skin, can have a special tightening effect (Gumbel 1993). Soothes insect bites and often added in insect-repellent blends, including for lice and scabies. Add to blends when sinuses are congested, especially with the feeling of "brain fog." Supports circulation, especially peripherally, protecting blood vessels and capillary health. Add to a synergy designed for muscle, joint, and tendon aches and pains, sprains, and bruises. Add to an abdominal massage blend (try with Roman chamomile and clary sage in a carrier) to relieve menstrual cramping.

- *Mentally:* Lemongrass's pleasant scent and anti-depressant components lighten mood, enabling clearer focus, cutting through the mental fog.
- *Emotionally:* Uplifting; associated with easing anxiety, depression, and being emotionally overwhelmed. Grief, insomnia, and times of transition, such as life changes, work, or living situations, may benefit from the "clearing" of lemongrass oil.
- *Spiritually:* As a grass, lemongrass is not soft: it is protective and as sharp as a paper's edge, allowing it to slice through the wind. Similarly, it can help cut through distractions of the mind and emotional heart, uplifting the body's responses to better health with confidence. The spirit always benefits when what is no longer needed can be removed and you have the freedom to let go, feeling protected, confident, and alive.

**Blends well with:** Basil, cedarwood, cypress, eucalyptus, ginger, laurel, lavender, lemon, palmarosa, patchouli, peppermint, rose geranium, rose, rosemary, sweet orange, ylang-ylang

**Precautions:** *Always, always dilute!* Lemongrass is very powerful and will cause dermal toxic reactions if used undiluted. This oil is *not* phototoxic, despite smelling like lemon, but it can be very irritating to the skin. Do not use more than 0.7% in a topical solution (no more than 5 drops in an ounce of carrier). Never use with children under 2 years of age, or with anyone who is hypersensitive or has damaged skin.

**Shelf life:** 2 to 3 years

# Palmarosa
*Soft—Powerful—Cooling*

**Common name:** Palmarosa

**Latin names:** *Cymbopogon martini* var. *motia* and its rarely used variation *Cymbopogon martini* var. *sofia*, commonly known as gingergrass

**Botanical family:** Poaceae, also called Graminaea, home as well to vetiver and lemongrass. Its genera comprise grass, rice, bamboo, sugar, and reeds, which grow all over the globe in various terrains, and produce 50 to 60 aromatic grasses.

**Attributes:** Cooling to the mind, heart, and body. Great for skin care and can be an uplifting addition to blends when you want a light rose-lemon scent.

**Character:** Has some similarities in appearance to its cousins vetiver and lemongrass: all grow in bunches and all are aromatic, but they are certainly different. As a tropical grass, grows well in humid environments; does best with well-drained, fertile, and organic matter in the mix. Does not tolerate frost and can be seeded during the monsoon seasons, hence its connection to water.

Its first year or two produces less essential oil, increasing by years three and four. Considered to be a productive crop for up to five years. Has been distilled since the 1700s. Due to its roselike aroma, has been used to adulterate precious rose oil; however, palmarosa has the additional bit of gentle citrus scent that a trained nose would be able to detect.

**Unique aroma:** Sweet, floral, roselike, soft, fresh, a bit of green, slightly citrusy-lemony, which can change depending on the country of origin and age of the oil

**Aromatic note:** Mid to top

**Part of plant used for essential oils:** Grass

**Countries of origin:** India, Southeast Asia, and Pakistan. The distilled oils come from India, Brazil, South Africa, and Nepal.

**Actions:** Antibacterial, anti-infectious, antifungal, anti-inflammatory, cellular rejuvenator, immunity regulator, neurotonic

**Uses:**

- *Physically:* Very good in antibacterial, antifungal, and antivirus blends. Add to a diffuser and personal inhalers for room and individual immunity-boosting, such as for colds, flu, bronchitis, and sinus issues. Supportive of skin cellular rejuvenation; a wonderful additional to mature or other skin preparations. Add to synergies to soothe skin that is dry or distressed, acne, eczema, psoriasis, or severe itching, and to smooth wrinkles. Its skin-regenerative capabilities will enhance blends used for cuts, abrasions, wounds, or broken capillaries in the skin. Because palmarosa has a soft cooling effect, dispelling excess heat, it can be used for fevers and excess sweating. Add to homemade deodorants. Effective in insect repellents. Use in diluted form for sitz baths and local washes; beneficial in blends or used alone for vaginitis, urethritis, and cystitis (Shutes 2015). Note: Only a doctor can diagnose these medical conditions, and if you have any of them, you should get your doctor's permission before you use palmarosa.

- *Mentally:* When the mind is calm, so shall the emotions and body reflect in kind. Clearing heat and invaders of the health of the body helps to clear the mind. This soft lemony-rose scent also taps into the potential of a softer way of thinking.

- *Emotionally:* Palmarosa's cooling attributes are good for hot emotions, nervous tension, stress, and irritability. Bring in when anxiety and nervousness invade the psyche; its aroma is great for easing the heart and soothing the emotions. Its cardio and neurotonic components aid the heart and emotions to find a more peaceful place to reside. Add to an evening blend, such as diffusing with neroli and lavender, to help quiet the mind and to relieve insomnia.

- *Spiritually:* In Ayurveda, the *ojas*, or vigor of the spirit, mind, emotions, and body, can be increased with consciously healthy choices. In Traditional Chinese Medicine, qi is the vital force within that flows and is renewable with, again, consciously healthy choices. Palmarosa feeds, nourishes, cools, and regenerates the vital health within the body, thus supporting the spirit. Add to meditation blends and when you need to connect to a sense of security, confidence, and love with yourself to set healthy boundaries and to make consciously healthy choices.

**Blends well with:** Cedarwood, frankincense, ginger, helichrysum, jasmine, laurel, lavender, lemongrass, niaouli, neroli, palo santo, patchouli, rosalina, rose geranium, rose, sandalwood, tea tree, vetiver

**Precautions:** This oil has a risk of mild skin sensitization, especially for sensitive individuals. It is much, much milder than its cousin lemongrass, and nice to add to many blends designed for skin regeneration and immunity boosting. However, keep the dilution level to 50 drops or less per ounce of carrier.

**Shelf life:** 4 to 5 years

## Skin Rejuvenation Blend

First, create a synergy in a ½-ounce amber or cobalt blue bottle:

3 drops palmarosa

2 drops helichrysum

3 drops lavender

3 drops frankincense or 1 drop patchouli

Then, add a carrier of your choice. Use on the body after a shower or when you have any skin concerns. Use a heavy carrier for dry skin needing extra nourishment, such as 80% jojoba/20% tamaru; or for normal skin, use jojoba, coconut, or almond carrier oils. This blend is great with apricot kernel oil for a lighter application that rubs in well.

Alternatively: For a facial oil, reduce the drops to 1 drop of each oil to equal 4 drops total. Then, you may adjust for scent by adding 2 more drops maximum. The total number of drops should not exceed 6 drops total for ½-ounce size facial oil.

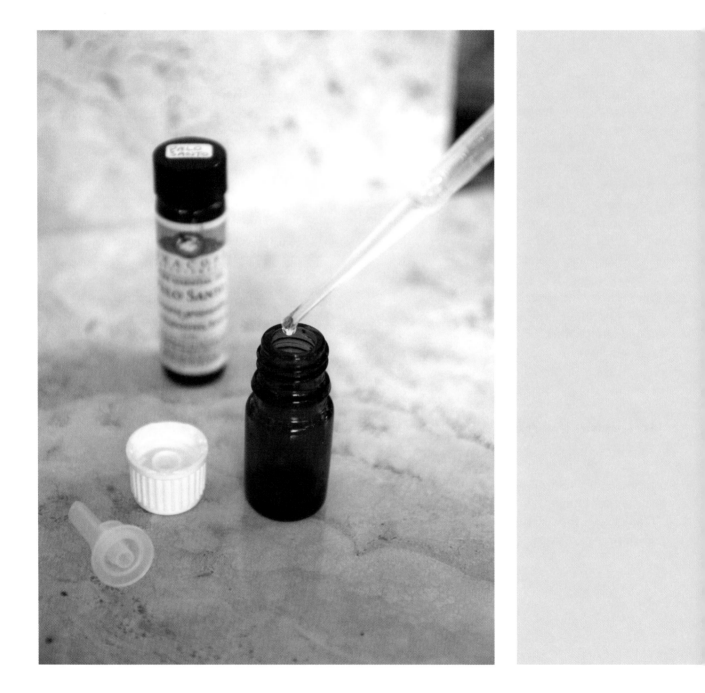

# Blends

**4**

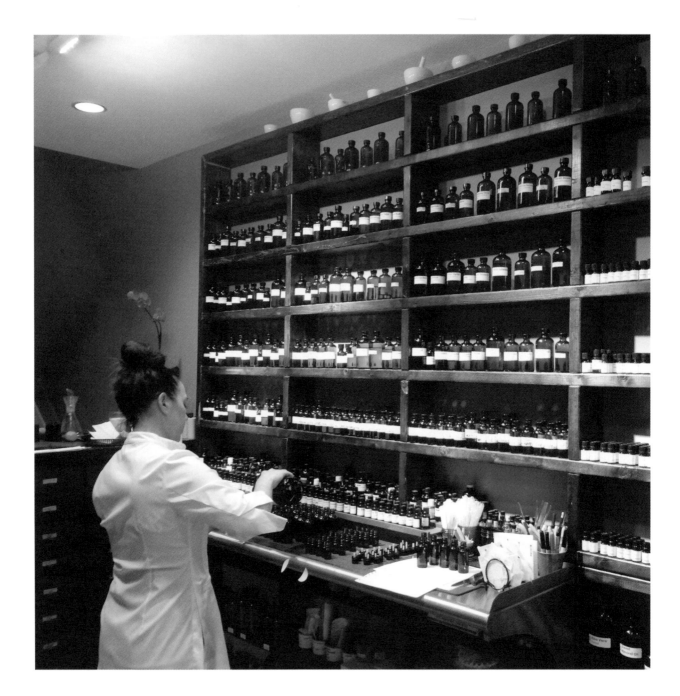

# CHAPTER 15

# Blending

*Coming together is a beginning; keeping together is progress;*
*working together is success.* —Henry Ford

Blending essential oils is an art all its own. How does someone who has created more than 60,000 custom blends bring it all together?

I had the privilege of shadowing clinical aromatherapist Theresa Cangialosi at her apothecary, Sobotanical. Apothecaries have traditionally been associated with pharmaceutical compounds using natural sources. In Theresa's shop, there are no synthetics. Instead, she sells natural soaps, essential oil diffusers, lotions, and other products that support stress relief and well-being. She is a master at using essential oils to assist the weary mind or heavy heart to find harmony. Her business is heavily based on custom blends for what a person needs at the time. She also has worked with the University of Maryland's Shock Trauma Center's Integrative Wellness program (see page 70) since 2012 and has created personalized blends for its many patients, including Richard Norris, recipient of the world's first full face transplant.

Watching Theresa blend a custom mix is a little like movie magic. A customer arrived, wanting a specific product, but didn't specify any particular smell or essential oils, trusting Theresa to do her thing. As she listened intently, I felt more than saw her process; it was as if the winds of wisdom deep within her stirred, rose up slowly around her, and swirled above her head—as if her essential oil and carrier options were themselves in consultation in the ether surrounding her. She then went into action to blend several oils in perfect harmony. Theresa then wrote down her custom recipe along with the person's name and filed it in a box along with the tens of thousands of creations she has made over the last 25 years or so. Her ability to blend well is what brings people back to her.

Of course, this was not a purely mystical experience. Theresa uses a combination of *logic* (what will make the most sense for a circumstance), *wisdom* (her knowledge of the essential oils them-

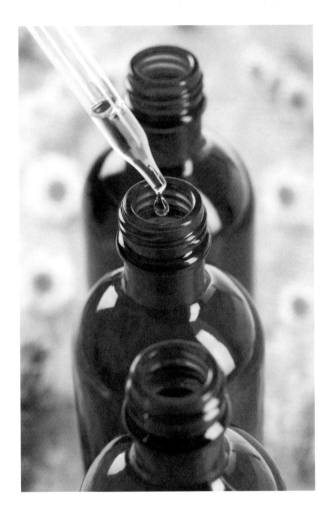

menting and it will help you have more successes than not.

Most people learn to blend in one or more of five ways:

1. **Description:** Get to know your oils by how they can best support you, such as whether they promote getting a better night's sleep or ease muscle soreness, by reading their complete profile (see Part 3).

2. **Scent:** Going by the oils' aroma is the most obvious, and by far the easiest, way to blend. But there is also a tricky side to scent—it changes! How an oil starts off may not be the same after 24 to 48 hours or even after 2 weeks! A great way to begin is to study the oils' entire profile, choose a few options for your intended purpose, and then narrow them down by scent.

3. **Recipe:** It can be very helpful to follow a step-by-step recipe when first creating synergies, blends, and combinations for specific purposes. This book offers numerous recipes to help you get started. Another version of a recipe is the 1-2-3 blending recipe: add 1 drop of a base note, 2 drops of a middle note, and 3 drops of a top note (the profiles in Part 3 identify these notes oil by oil). This is a fun, easy way to create blends, plus it teaches you how to distinguish among top, mid, and base notes.

selves, safety guidelines, and what has worked in the past), and *intuition* (what the person needs but is not able to express in words). If you start, like Theresa, with a mindful plan of which oils are appropriate for your blends and purpose, you won't waste your precious essential oils experi-

4. **Intuition:** Using your intuition comes with time, practice, and willingness to follow the lead of the essential oils. In the beginning, I would set out a group of essential oils that met the descriptions I was looking for, but then something would happen . . . it was as if the best essential oils for my purpose called to me for that blend. You may also have an instinctual feeling that a particular oil is just right for a particular person. But be mindful; your intuition may be correct, but you need to pair this information with knowing as much as you can about the oils that call to you as well as discussing with recipients what they believe to be their needs, especially if you are not a practitioner, or certified or clinical aroma-therapist. Safety always applies.

5. **Chemistry:** This is the most advanced method and really only comes after years of experience and training. Once you know the chemical com-ponents of specific essential oils, you can find the exact constituents that meet your needs. For instance, if you are looking for something with high monoterpenes, you can narrow down your list with oils with those components. I only men-tion it here for aspiring aromatherapists who wish to do further study.

You do not have to be proficient in all five areas to be great at blending; some people do best at just one or two of these approaches and that's okay! Remember, your goals are to provide stress relief and do no harm.

## Dosage

The best way to use essential oils safely is to use the appropriate dosages in your blends. The "Basic Dosage" chart on page 226 is the best way to make sure you do this, and the conversion chart a little further on will help you measure the right dosages with non-metric measurements. (All the charts in this chapter have been compiled with permission from Jade Shutes and with Tisserand and Young's dilution safety recommendations for general use, with permission of Elsevier.)

### DROP BY DROP

Each drop of an essential oil contains the botani-cal wisdom and chemical matrix of its parent plant. Each combination you create will have a particular number of drops of each essential oil that you are using. The challenge here is that there is no exact measurement of a drop. How big a "drop" is depends on what device the oil is dropping from, and how big that device's opening is, and sometimes on the heaviness of the oil itself.

Since it is hard to pinpoint an exact drop mea-surement, professionals estimate the number of drops per milliliter (or other volume), allowing for the variables just mentioned. Robert Tisserand says a milliliter could comprise anywhere from 20 to 40 drops, so he uses an average of 30 drops, taking into consideration the size of the drop. (If the drops are bigger, there will be fewer drops per milliliter.) Andrea Butje, owner of Aromahead

Institute, says she has found the average milliliter holds between 18 and 45 drops, so she teaches her students to use an average of 25 drops per milliliter (2017). For the purposes of getting you started on learning drop potency, I have assumed that one milliliter comprises an average of 30 drops. If in doubt, always measure conservatively and use fewer drops of essential oil.

The "Basic Dosage" chart (page 226) tells you the total number of drops to use in a particular quantity of carrier oil to achieve a specific dilution. The total number of drops can be of one essential oil or a combination of different essential oils, as long as the total number of drops of essential oils does not exceed the total number of drops listed. For instance, to achieve a 1% dilution in 1 ounce of carrier oil, you can safely add up to nine drops of essential oil—say, three drops each of three different essential oils or nine drops of one essential oil—but not nine drops each of multiple essential oils.

Another factor that may affect how many drops of essential oil you need is the size of the opening of the essential oil bottle you're using. Most essential oil bottles come with orifice reducers on the top: the hard plastic top has a small opening that allows only one drop of oil to come out at a time. But not all orifice reducers are equal. Some companies use larger orifice reducers that create bigger drops. Using oil from a bottle with a larger orifice reducer could cause you to add too much essential oil to blends, especially for special groups that need less, not more, essential oil, such as children

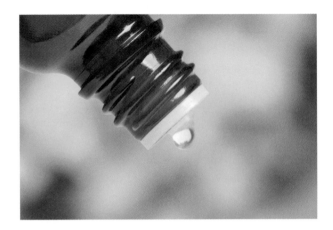

and the elderly. On the other hand, smaller bottles, such as bottles that are the size of a fluid dram (1/16 ounce), tend to have very small openings (I sometimes call them mini-drops).

The only way to create consistency in your drop size is to use a pipette, which is a tube designed for releasing fluids by the drop. Pipettes can easily be purchased online in large packages. (I get mine in a pack of 100.) But be careful: You can use each pipette only once, for one essential oil. If you use a pipette for more than one essential oil, you will end up with cross contamination—eeek! No matter how careful you are, a minute amount of essential oil will always be left within the pipette that cannot be used to create your blend. Spent pipettes can be placed in a glass jar to use as a room scent while it lasts.

One last variable in getting your essential oil out of its bottle is that some oils are more viscous than others. Citrus oils tend to come out of the bot-

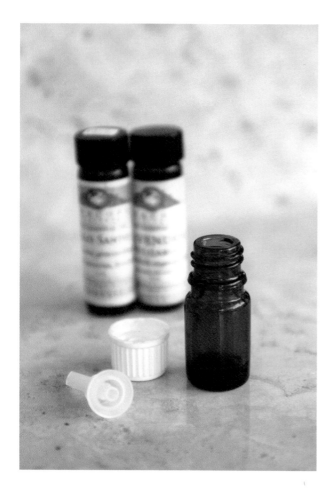

tle fairly quickly, whereas vetiver is a superthick oil that teaches you about patience, grounding, and learning to pause while you wait for that one single drop to finally emerge. (Really, vetiver is in no hurry. Keep this in mind when blending for someone who does not know how to find stillness.)

Synergies and blends usually have a window of how many drops can be added to a certain dilution. Use the *least* amount of drops first, so you have some room to make adjustments if necessary. If extra drops fall in when you're counting, do not worry; just add them to the overall count (write it down!) and move on. Be mindful of your overall count. For example, a 1-ounce bottle of carrier at 2% dilution has a window of 12 to 18 drops. Start out aiming for the 12 drops, and then you can use the extra drops to adjust for scent or for circumstances that allow for the maximum in that percentage, in this case 18 drops.

If working with children or teens, use the lower number in the recommended window of drops; likewise, if a person is health compromised in any way and needs a gentler approach. Always think "Safety first" and "Less is more"; you want to aim for creating *less* stress in the body.

## Basic Dosage

| DILUTION PERCENTAGE | DROPS PER 10 ML (0.25 OZ) CARRIER | DROPS PER 15 ML (0.5 OZ) CARRIER | DROPS PER 20 ML (0.75 OZ) CARRIER | DROPS PER 30 ML (1 OZ) CARRIER | DROPS PER 45 ML (1.5 OZ) CARRIER | DROPS PER 60 ML (2.0 OZ) CARRIER |
|---|---|---|---|---|---|---|
| 0.5% | 1 | 2 | 2–3 | 3–4 | 5–7 | 6–8 |
| 1% | 3 | 3–4 | 5–6 | 7–9 | 10–15 | 15–18 |
| 2% | 4–6 | 7–9 | 10–12 | 12–18 | 22–30 | 30–36 |
| 2.5% | 7–8 | 10–11 | 14–16 | 20–22 | 36–38 | 43–46 |
| 3% | 8–9 | 12–13 | 16–18 | 25–27 | 40–45 | 48–54 |
| 4% | 10–12 | 15–18 | 20–24 | 30–36 | 55–60 | 68–72 |
| 5% | 13–15 | 20–22 | 28–30 | 40–45 | 70–75 | 78–90 |

## Dilution and Percentages

Dilution is how you create a safe blend. The term *dilution* is the concentration of a substance within the base substance. Aromatherapists refer to *percentages* to give a ratio of essential oil to carrier in a fast way, with an understanding that within their recommended window, the number of drops could vary a tad but the overall amount is controlled. That is, they will often say a product has a 1% dilution, rather than how many drops it contains, because 1% is the potency in a 1-ounce bottle as well as in a 4-ounce bottle.

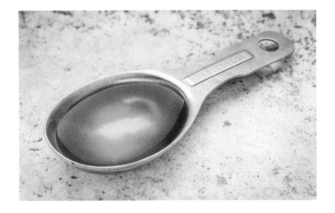

## Conversion Chart

| AVERAGE NUMBER OF DROPS (APPROXIMATE WINDOW) | MILLILITERS | OUNCES | TEASPOONS | TABLESPOONS |
|---|---|---|---|---|
| 30 (20–40) | 1 | 0.03 | 0.2 | 0.07 |
| 150 (100–200) | 5 | 0.17 | 1 | 0.34 |
| 210 (140–280) | 7 | 0.25 | 1.5 | 0.5 |
| 300 (200–400) | 10 | 0.34 | 2 | 0.7 |
| 450 (300–600) | 15 | 0.5 | 3 | 1 |
| 900 (600–1,200) | 30 | 1 | 6 | 2 |

When looking at the "Basic Dosage" chart, take note that dilution is in direct proportion to the *liquid volume* of carrier being used, not the *kind* of carrier. A 1-ounce bottle of carrier oil takes the same dilution as 1 ounce of unscented lotion. That is, the percentage does not change if the base (oil, lotion, etc.) changes. The percentage of concentration changes only if the *amount* of the base changes, say, from 1 ounce to 2 ounces.

It is very common for milliliters to be used instead of ounces, so both are given for your convenience as well as to familiarize you with standard conversions: 1 fluid ounce equals approximately 30 ml. For true accuracy, amount would be measured by weight using a digital scale.

In the "Basic Dosage" chart, the measurements are *approximate*, based on an *average* number of drops per milliliter. As noted earlier, depending on the liquid and the size of a drop and the orifice reducer or pipette used, a "drop" can be larger or smaller. Consider this when measuring. These conversions are based on an average of 30 drops per ml.

## HOW TO DILUTE ESSENTIAL OILS PROPERLY

Dilutions are recommended based on several factors: age of user, intended use, how often it will be applied, and whether the issue is acute or chronic. It is important to follow the recommended charts when you begin blending. Essential oils are natural botanical resources that the body recognizes and adjusts to accordingly, so it is not necessary to jump to a higher percentage or dilution unless indicated. In fact, if blends are too potent or used too frequently, the body may respond with an irritation, allergic reaction, or sensitization. To

## Recommended Dilution Rate by Purpose

| DILUTION RATE | PURPOSES AND INDICATORS | DROPS PER 1 OZ (30 ML) OF CARRIER |
|---|---|---|
| 0.25–0.5% | Frail/elderly individuals, irritated or sensitive skin | 1–2 drops max |
| 1% | Pregnancy, face creams | 7–9 drops max |
| 1–4% | Bath and body products | 7–36 drops max |
| up to 1.5% | Subtle aromatherapy, emotional and energetic work, pregnancy, frail/elderly, face cream and lotions, facial cosmetics, exfoliate, oily skin | 10 drops max |
| 2–5% | Nervous system, well-being, daily stress, endocrine system, general massage, general skin care, massage oils, lotions, face oils, body oils, body butters, general holistic approaches (2.5%) | 12–45 drops max |
| 4–10% | Specific problems (local problems; e.g., muscle or menstrual pains). Note: the higher the percentage, the more localized the area (think spot treatment). | 30–60 drops max |

avoid this possibility, refer to the "Basic Dosage" and follow charts and keep written notes on blends you try, create, and may need for the future.

Although essential oils are natural botanical components, remember that this does not make them biocompatible—that is, compatible with your biology—in their pure form. Used all by themselves, they tend to be drying, strong, and are more attracted to lipids (*lipophilic*) than waters (*hydrophobic*). The human body is mostly water. Hence, dilution in a carrier gives the oils something wonderful to connect to as a means to interact safely and effectively with a human body. You will learn more about this in the next chapter, but for now, keep in mind that oils' relationship with an appropriate carrier is intimately related to their use and safety.

### ESSENTIAL OILS AND CHILDREN

We've already noted that essential oils are powerful, active substances. Before you use any essential oils on or around children, consult with a pediatrician and qualified aromatherapist. Also, consider whether there may be methods other than essential oils to alleviate the problem you're trying to solve, such as a change in routine, food, rest, compresses, humidifiers, herbs, or a doctor appointment.

If you do end up using essential oils on or around children, please remember:

## Recommended Dilution by Age For Children

Note: Always get pediatrician's approval for use of essential oils with infants and children. In addition, consult with a trained aromatherapist for contraindications and proper use.

| AGE | DILUTION PERCENTAGE | DROPS PER 1 OZ (30 ML) OF CARRIER |
|---|---|---|
| Premature babies | DO NOT USE | DO NOT USE |
| Up to 3 months | | Hydrosol mist in the air, spray, or diluted in humidifier—use only if necessary. |
| Up to 3 months | 0.1–0.2% | 1–2 drops max in a full ounce of carrier—use only if necessary; unscented carriers may be best up to 24 months for some babies. Consult a trained aromatherapist. |
| 3–24 months | 0.25–0.5% | 2–4 drops max—always start with the lowest number of drops. |
| 2–6 years | 1–2% | 8–18 drops max |
| 6–15 years | 1.5–3% | 12–28 drops max |
| 15 or older | 2.5–5% | 22–45 drops max |

- Dilute. Dilute. Dilute. Always check the chart "Recommended Dilution by Age for Children" for appropriate dilutions. (See page 271 for bath time dilution suggestions.)
- Never let a child ingest essential oils in any shape or form.
- Do not use blends with children. Introduce one essential oil at a time at proper dilution. Consult an aromatherapist before using any blends with older children, including any commercial or private proprietary blends. Some blends are not kid-safe.
- Do not use essential oils every day with children. They do not need it. Children are very sensitive. Use these wonderful tools only when a situation warrants use.
- Rotate essential oils that you use with children.
- Always be observant of how your child is reacting to essential oils: keep an eye on both their skin and their mood.
- It is best to introduce essential oils in a room diffuser, rather than using the oils topically. If you use a diffuser, run it for no more than 10 to 15 minutes at a time for young kids and up to 30 minutes for older children and teens, turning off for 1 to 2 hours before running again. Do not run a diffuser all night—it is far too much essential oil for children (or adults!) to metab-

## Hydrosols Generally Considered Safe for Children
Note: Always get pediatrician's approval and consult a qualified aromatherapist.

| HYDROSOL | PURPOSE | USES |
|---|---|---|
| Chamomile | Rest, calming, antibacterial, scrapes, diaper rash | Room mists, diluted 25% to full strength.<br><br>Add 1/4–1/2 cup to humidifier water. Use instead of essential oils in a room diffuser.<br><br>Add 1/4 teaspoon up to 2 teaspoons in 1 cup of water for digestive upsets.<br><br>Use in the summertime to cool down hot children. Use instead of water in compresses (with adults, too!). |
| Lavender | Rest, calming, antibacterial, skin, diaper rash | |
| Helichrysum | Skin, diaper rash | |
| Fennel | Gas, bloating | |
| Neroli | Rest, calming | |
| Frankincense | Rest, antibacterial, skin, diaper rash | |
| Rose | Calming, rest, skin | |

olize and could lead to sensitization due to overexposure.

*Caution*: Eucalyptus and peppermint require very specific safety considerations when used with children (including strong restrictions and contra-indications), especially for the very young. Consult with an aromatherapist for proper, safe usage with these oils, individually as well as in any blends.

## ESSENTIAL OILS AND PREGNANCY
In the very special months a woman spends in pregnancy, and the time frame of breastfeeding, consideration and care must be taken when using essential oils. Many oils simply are best avoided during this time. It is much easier to keep essential oil use to a minimum, and use under the guidance of an aromatherapist. Remember, too, that each woman may respond to scent very differently during pregnancy.

Inhalation of ginger, sweet orange, or lavender may be pleasing as well as reduce sensations of nausea. An important essential oil best avoided during pregnancy, but that can be used to assist labor, is clary sage.

Common essential oils that should be avoided all together during pregnancy and breastfeeding are birch, carrot seed, fennel, Spanish lavender, myrrh, oregano, and wintergreen. (Additionally, some others—associated more with clinical aromatherapy—that should also be avoided during pregnancy and breastfeeding include anise, cassia, cinnamon bark, feverfew, mugwort, rue, pennyroyal, tansy, worm-wood, and yarrow.) For a good list of essential oils to avoid during pregnancy and lactation, I suggest consulting *Essential Oil Safety*, 2nd ed., by Robert Tisserand and Rodney Young, pages 152–53.

## Top, Mid, and Base Notes

Every synergy and blend is meant to do one of two things: provide comfort or stimulate action. *Comfort* can soothe the worried mind or anxious heart. It can also relax the body for a good night's rest, or simply create a desirable atmosphere in a room. To *stimu-late* is to move molecules to do something in partic-ular, such as to liquefy mucus so it can be expelled easier or reduce inflammation in a stressed muscle. Ultimately, these functions prompt the vital forces within your body to support well-being.

When creating a synergy, it is best to place your essential oils together in a glass bottle, gently swirl them, and then take a sniff. You want to check in with the communication between these wonderful oils as they move into a bonded relationship. I first learned this method from perfumer and aromather-apist Shannon Metcalf as a means to observe scent relationships, rather than "just mixing." Does one component smell more strongly than another? Is there one you wish you could pick up a little more? It can be helpful to know what is happening with your sniff test before blending with a carrier scent.

Several things are happening in a synergy. First, the oils are combining to create something new. Second, they are maintaining their own personal integrity while they do so. As they become more familiar with one another and the relationship devel-ops, the scent will begin to change over time. This is due to the oils' volatile nature, their individual mass (heaviness), and their ability to phytochemi-cally bond. Synergies can change over a matter of minutes, but the real test is what happens during the span of 24 hours to 2 weeks. Think of a really good spaghetti sauce: Individual ingredients are put into a pot and then simmered for several hours. The flavors come together, producing a sauce of complexity, yet no one flavor stands out above the rest. This is your goal when creating a synergy and later a blend: no one essential oil outshining the others is the sign of a good relationship.

If you are using blends topically, you might notice that the scent changes in connection with your own biological influences. Sometimes the blend in the bottle will smell different after an hour on your body! This is often due to the relationship between the essential oils' exposure to the air and their absorption into your body.

Another consideration is what is known as dry out. It tests how much of an aroma remains after the most volatile compounds (those that vaporize the fastest), have dissipated and the heavier molecules are left to stabilize the scent. Dry out is best done using a paper test strip (you can order them for your own home use). If you do not have the perfumers' test strips, use a thick, preferably natural, acid-free, white strip of paper. Cardstock will work in a pinch.

Drop a single drop of essential oil on the strip and expose it to the air. You can do this by securing it to stand up, holding it with your hand, or letting it suspend over the edge of a surface, such as a counter, so air can circulate all around the strip. This will show you how quickly an oil evaporates and also how its aromatic qualities change over time.

As time passes, an oil emits three different layers of fragrance:

- *Top note:* The first and lightest aromatic molecules to evaporate from the essential oil. These give the first smells in a blend and do not last as long as a mid or base note. These oils tend to oxidize very easily due to their ability to quickly mix with the air (think: little bubbles popping at the surface in an effervescent drink).

- *Mid note:* The next layer of vapors to leave an essential oil. These take longer to evaporate, tend to be slower to oxidize, and can carry a blend a little longer due to the propensity to linger a bit before changing form. There is a wide range of mid notes that help bridge and bind the top and base together (think: the bubbles that cling to the side of a glass for a long time before rising to the surface).

- *Base note:* The deep notes of a blend that are often used as a fixative to "fix" a top or mid note and so help the aroma last longer. Base notes are often thick oils, earthy in fragrance, and by themselves have a heavier, slower pulse than the fast hummingbird beat of a top note. Base notes usually have longer shelf lives and act as grounding agents spiritually and emotionally (think: the body of an effervescent liquid that remains still once the bubbles go up to the top).

## Fragrance Intensity

Top, mid, and base notes are different from *fragrance intensity*, which is what perfumers use to identify how *strong* an aroma is, not how quickly it vaporizes. For instance, a strong essential oil with a high fragrance intensity, such as Roman chamomile and vetiver, requires fewer drops in a blend because it smells stronger. For essential oils with highly volatile properties (they evaporate more quickly) that are considered top notes, more drops can be added, as is the case with sweet orange, whose fragrance will be drowned out easily by the intense aromas of vetiver or patchouli.

bergamot, lavender, rose geranium, or clary sage. You might also add a bit of palmarosa, ylang-ylang, jasmine, neroli, sandalwood, or cedarwood. For blends that need something to bridge between a few already strong odors, try marjoram, orange, mandarin, neroli, bergamot, ylang-ylang, jasmine, geranium, or rose or rose-scented essential oils (Rhind 2012).

## Smoothing Out Your Synergy

Occasionally, you will create a really great synergy, but for some reason, the oils are just missing that certain ooh-la-la to help them harmonize. Try a drop or two of sweet marjoram. Do not add so much that the overall aroma changes to smelling like marjoram; rather, allow marjoram to bridge the two worlds to meet. Let nature find itself within the bottle gently; it won't take much. Swirl the new mixture gently and smell. Sometimes lavender can help harmonize a blend, but be mindful—add too much and it will smell like lavender. Ho wood, another harmonizer, adds a soft "powdery" element. Other essences often used to smooth out a blend in perfumery act as scents that either "hold down" the top notes from flying away or add a bit of lightness to a mix. Use sparingly (1 drop is often all that is needed, no more) when smoothing out a blend. To add personality, try patchouli, peppermint, or one of the chamomiles. To round out a synergy with the intention of adding a bit of scent, try lemon,

## Supplies for Blending

- *Glass jars or bottles:* Amber (brown) or cobalt (blue) help keep light out of the container. Wide-mouth jars are great for lotions, creams, and rubs. For small quantities of your oil creations, use smaller jars or bottles appropriate to the product. The less air in the container, the better. In most cases, there is no need to create more than an ounce of a blend while you are learning.
- *Pipettes,* for controlled drops while measuring
- *Pen or pencil and a notebook or recipe book* to write down all your creations. Leave room to document what you did or did not like about a blend after it has "settled" a bit (usually within 24 hours to 2 weeks). I have small notes of "what I learned in making this" next to some of mine, along with "what I would change next time."
- *Glass stir rod or nonreactive metal spoon* (you can use the handle) to stir your base and synergy together (do not use plastic)

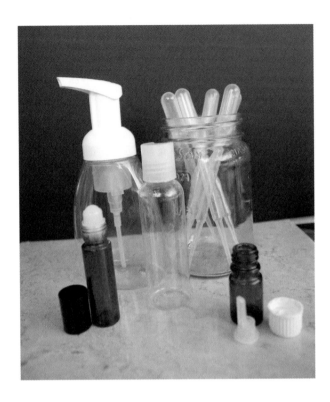

before you start working, too. Works great for linen sprays, too. Vodka is sometimes used if 190 proof is unavailable. Do not use rubbing alcohol.

- *Unscented lotion or cream*
- *Liquid soap, shampoo, full-fat milk or cream, or salt* for a bath blend (you can use Epsom salts, Himalayan pink salt, Dead Sea salt, sea salt, or a combination); baking soda optional
- *Filtered or distilled water* for diffusers
- *Carrier oils*
- *Aloe vera gel*
- *Hydrosols*
- *Gloves* for safety and cleanliness

## Blending Basics

Ikebana, the Japanese art of flower arranging, brings all the elements of nature into account: the individual shapes and forms of branches, flowers, leaves, and stems as well as the container itself. No item is overlooked or placed without purpose and intention. Harmony, simplicity, and beauty are key to this style of flower arrangement. And so it is when creating a synergy or a blend using essential oils.

- *Have a purpose.* Decide whether you are designing for pleasure or to assist with physical, emotional, mental, or spiritual support.
- *Pick your medium.* Are you going to use an oil carrier, cream, lotion, or gel base? Or are you mak-

- *PET containers:* These are acceptable (and sometimes a better option than glass) for certain products (e.g., for travel or hand or face washes).
- *Roller bottles:* These have a ball atop an amber or cobalt blue glass bottle that enables you to apply roll-ons (great for those unfamiliar with essential oils).
- *Personal inhalers (a.k.a. aromawands or aromasticks):* Use on the go, anywhere, anytime.
- *Alcohol,* to sterilize your clean containers before using—190 proof alcohol. It evaporates quickly and is great for countertop areas

ing a hand or facial soap or bath salt? Or are you going to disperse in a diffuser? Keep it simple for yourself and the person who will be using the product.

- *Pick your oils.* Your purpose will be a big help in deciding on which oils to use. When starting, limit yourself to using no more than three essential oils at a time. You can build more complex synergies later (and you will, because it is fun and loveliness can be made with five oils or more). But do not go overboard; be mindful, be gentle. Little ones and those with a compromised system might require that use of no more than one oil at a time.

- *Synergy first.* If blending two or more oils together, it is best to place them in your desired container first and then add the carrier. This allows you to check the smell first and to make small adjustments. Plus, it allows the essential oils to create a relationship before being blended with the carrier. Drop a few oils into the bottom of the container you will be using, then gently swirl or roll it between both of your hands. It won't take much to get it going. This is preferable to rapidly shaking. Think: synergy; think: bringing together. Invite the oils to join one another, rather than forcefully combining them.

Let's create a couple of examples and then you can experiment more (see Chapter 17) after reading about your carrier choices.

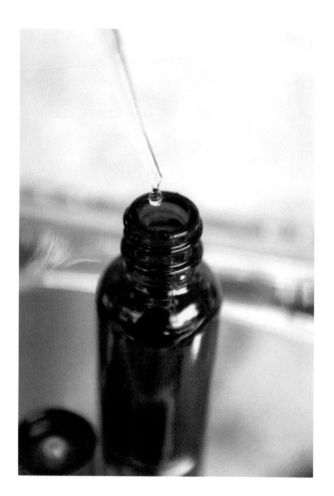

## Sunshine Zest

**Purpose:** Uplift the energy feel and mood in the room
**Medium:** Diffuser
**Essential Oils:** *Citrus:* Reduces stress and anxiety, and has a calming effect on the nervous system
*Ginger:* Adds a nice warm and spicy aroma to the mix; stimulates energy

*Piñon pine*: Purifies air, encourages deep breathing

**Synergy:** No need to mix the oils first unless creating a synergy to keep and use later. Combine:

2 to 3 drops mandarin, grapefruit, or sweet orange
1 drop ginger
1 drop piñon pine

1.  Pour an appropriate amount of water up to the fill line of your diffuser (do not go over the fill line; mine holds approximately ⅓ cup of water). Add the essential oils directly to the water.

2.  Run the diffuser for 30 to 60 minutes on, then turn off for at least 30 to 60 minutes. For children, only run for 10 to 20 minutes, then turn off for at least an hour or two.

## Nighttime Foot Love (spring and summer)

**Purpose:** End-of-day relaxing foot rub

**Medium:** Unscented lotion or cream

**Essential Oils:** *Lavender*: Assists with insomnia and sleep disorders, relaxing, sedative

*Rose geranium*: Relaxing, cooling, soothes the nervous system

*Patchouli*: Good for insomnia, grounding, centering

**Synergy:** In a clean, empty 2-ounce PET jar/container, combine (35 drops total for a 2.5% solution):

15 drops lavender
12 drops rose geranium
8 drops patchouli

1.  Create the synergy first in the container. Gently roll around to harmonize before adding the carrier to the jar. Tip: You might find it a little bit easier to add a little carrier, then use your stir stick to mix the oils as much as you can before adding a little more carrier at a time. It can be challenging to add all the carrier to a small container and not have much mixing room (it tends to fall out of the container while you are trying to mix up everything at the bottom).

2.  Close lid and label the ingredients, date, and the name of the item.

3.  Rub on clean feet up to 30 minutes before going to sleep, massaging the entire bottom and top of your feet. Rub any leftover mixture into your hands and/or chest, and last, run your hands through your hair. Any tiny bit left on your hands will lightly scent your hair without heavy residue.

## Dry Skin Nourish (women, mature skin, fall, winter)

**Purpose:** To soothe dry mature skin for women during the fall and winter months (body only, not face)

**Medium:** Massage oil blend of 50% sweet almond oil, 30% jojoba oil, and 20% calendula herbal oil

**Essential Oils:** *Clary sage*: Harmonizing, soothing, reassuring

*Rose geranium*: Relaxing, cooling, soothes the nervous system

*Helichrysum*: Skin healing

**Synergy:** In a clean, empty 1-ounce glass jar/container, combine (18 drops total for a 2.5% dilution):

6 drops clary sage

6 drops rose geranium

6 drops helichrysum

1. Create the synergy first in the container. Gently roll or swirl around to harmonize before adding the carrier oils to the container. Slowly add enough sweet almond oil to go to the halfway point on the bottle. Yes, you will be eyeballing this, so try to look at the bottle from the side and not from above, to watch the fill line. In the remaining headspace of the bottle, go just past halfway with jojoba. Last, fill the remaining space just up to the neckline (right where the bottle changes shape to the neck) with calendula herbal oil.

2. Close the lid; gently roll and rotate between both of your hands for several minutes. Open to smell the new blend.

3. Label with the name of the blend, date, and ingredients.

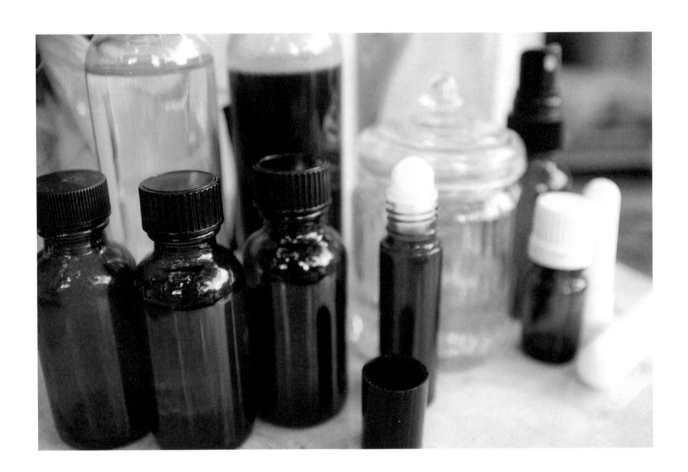

# CHAPTER 16

# Carrier Oils

*Just as food eaten without appetite is a tedious nourishment, so does study without zeal damage the memory by not assimilating what it absorbs.* —Leonardo da Vinci

Carrier oils carry the essential oil over larger areas of the body as well as into the skin. I prefer to think of them as nutrient bases. These amazing oils are often underestimated in regards to their intrinsic value. Carriers are not simply an elevator ride to the deeper skin levels, where the door opens and essential oils step off. Carriers are luscious, nutritive rich, aromatic, colorful, and sensual to the touch. They can be warming or cooling, slippery, slick, viscous, or light and absorbent. They are also referred to as "fixed oils" due to their nonvolatile nature (they do not vaporize like essential oils).

Carriers are not limited to oils, however. Lotions and creams are a blend of oils and water. Butters are thick and luxurious, not as easily absorbed into the skin, great for massage or dry skin. Gel bases, such as those with soothing, cooling aloe vera, aid heat-related issues, such as sunburns and wound heal-ing. Soaps are temporary carriers as they are easily washed off; they are used more like scent holders rather than skin-delivery systems. Dry salts mixed with carrier oils allow essential oils to be trans-formed into available physical, emotional, mental, and spiritual soothers.

The more nutrient rich a carrier is, the more fra-grant it will be; it will also be more deeply colored. The increased aroma as well as the color sometimes contribute beautifully to a blend. But while creating your own blends, always ask yourself: will it be used therapeutically or for pleasure? Appropriate sup-portive components for a particular issue should be considered first when creating a physically therapeu-tic blend; its scent is secondary (although primary with mental and emotional concerns). In some cases a blend may need to be harmonized with a less aro-matic oil, such jojoba.

In her webinar, Rose Chard explains that no matter whether you are using essential oils for therapeutic purposes or not, the therapeutics of the nutritive-rich fixed oils will benefit the overall health of the skin regardless of how much essential oil is penetrated into the skin (2016). Meanwhile, Robert Tisserand reminds us that the absorption rate through the skin is lower than inhalation. The intention of use is important; for instance, a sore muscle will gain greater benefit with massage with essential oils than through inhalation of essential oils alone (2016).

Carrier oils are composed mostly (85 to 99%) of lipids, which are a combination of fatty acids, many of which contain nutritive aspects humans can utilize for health. The remaining components (1 to 15%) give the carrier its aroma, color, taste, and individual personality. Some lipids are in constant liquid form (unsaturated); others become solid when cooled, and others are mostly solid like butters (saturated). Here is a list of some of the most basic lipids found in carrier oils, and their therapeutic uses.

(The following information has been compiled from Jade Shutes [2016], Susan M. Parker [2014], and Rose Chard [2016].)

## ALPHA LINOLENIC ACID (ALA, OMEGA-3)

- Not synthesized by the human body, so must be taken in from an outside source
- Absorbs into the skin quickly
- Converts into two compounds found in fish oils
- Anti-inflammatory
- Protects circulatory system
- Relieves itching, redness, and irritation of skin
- Found in seeds
- *Carrier oils high in ALA*: red raspberry, walnut, blackberry, chia, and flaxseed

## LINOLEIC ACID (LA, OMEGA-6)

- Not synthesized by the human body, so must be taken in from an outside source
- Builds the membrane that surrounds every skin cell
- Strengthens and protects the lipid barrier just beneath the skin surface
- Guards against moisture loss
- Keeps dirt, bacteria, and outside chemicals from entering the skin
- Absorbs quickly into the skin
- Deficiencies are often related to acne or scaly skin and dryness
- Converts to gamma linoleic acid (GLA)
- *Carrier oils high in LA*: grapeseed, safflower, evening primrose, passionfruit seed

## GAMMA LINOLEIC ACID (GLA)

- An omega-6 fatty acid, derived from linoleic acid
- Anti-inflammatory
- Soothes red, itchy, irritated skin
- Helps maintain moisture

- Supports skin barrier functions
- Assists with conditions such as eczema, psoriasis, dermatitis, and rheumatoid arthritis
- Aids in wound healing
- Deficiencies include signs of rough, dry, cracked skin that is easily bruised, tendencies toward eczema, and fragile and dull hair
- *Carrier oils high in GLA*: borage seed oil, black currant, evening primrose

## OLEIC ACID (OMEGA-9)

- Most common fatty acid found in vegetable oils (also in animal fats)
- Good for already healthy skin; maintains stability in health
- Produced by sebum in the body
- "If linoleic acid is deficient in the skin, oleic acid can make the problem worse by increasing sebum production" (Parker 2014). That is, use only on already healthy skin.
- Help resist damaging effects of heat and light
- Supports skin barrier functions
- *Carrier oils high in oleic acid*: macadamia, camellia, hazelnut, almond, avocado, marula, moringa, olive

Do keep in mind that scent always matters. Even though therapeutics sometimes take center stage, if the user does not like the scent, or if it is too intense, then no matter how great its benefits, the product likely will end up ignored, hidden, or thrown away. That said, people may be willing to

> ### BEWARE OF CLEAR, ODORLESS OILS
>
> Commercially sold oils have been processed to be as clear and scentless as possible, suggesting purity, and to extend their shelf life. "Waxes and scent and color are removed to create oils that are uniform for the market, ship and store well in all weather, and keep them from going rancid too quickly. This is the uninteresting pale vegetable oil found on grocery shelves," writes Susan M. Parker, author of *Power of the Seed: Your Guide to Oils for Health & Beauty*. This is common practice in the manufacture of cosmetics. Select genuinely pure carriers that still contain their natural nutrients; nutrient-stripped processed oils provide little therapeutic benefit.

give something new and different a try if they know it will help. I think of this as teaching the body, brain, and sense of smell how to identify and appreciate unfamiliar helpers. (Think of herbal medicines that taste bad but got the job done.) Use your own judgment and ask for feedback on scent sensitivity with yourself and others (remember, scent can be incredibly different from one person to the next). Bottom line: stress relief with essential oils must maintain harmony between the user and the product.

# How to Choose a Carrier

Knowing how and why you intend to apply essential oils will help determine which carrier is suitable, be it an oil, lotion, cream, salve, gel, or water, or whether to find an appropriate hydrosol instead.

**Carrier oils** work best for massage. They can be used for facial oils and for large areas of the body, any time of the year, are fine for all ages, and are complementary to mature skin. Some, such as sesame, are known for their warming feel; others, such as coconut, for their cooling nature. Thicker oils as such will be slower to absorb, whereas lighter oils absorb fairly quickly and may be thin enough to work in roller ball applications. Carrier oils are especially nice for dry, cold winter months. (*Caution:* Do not use carrier oils to treat fungus; use gel bases instead.)

Carrier oils can be mixed together; for instance, I have mixed a little each of jojoba and apricot kernel oil together as my base and added essential oils. Some oils are a better match than others, so play with a few starter oils and notice how they *feel* to you, on your fingers and on your body. Each body will also play a part in the relationship of the carrier oil.

**Herbal infused oils**, sometimes called macerated oils, are base oils, usually olive, in which herbs and plants have been infused. The ingredients harmonize for several weeks in a sealed jar, imparting a synergy, often fueled by natural sunlight. The plant material is then strained out, leaving behind a plant-

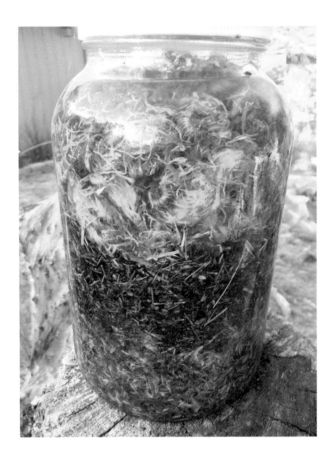

oil energy. Making flavored, scented, and medicinal oils have been processed this way throughout cultures and for thousands of years.

**Lotions and creams** make wonderful carriers for essential oils and are supereasy to use, especially all over the body, in massage, or for foot and hand applications; they feel nice to the touch and rub in well. Lotions and creams are well suited for warmer

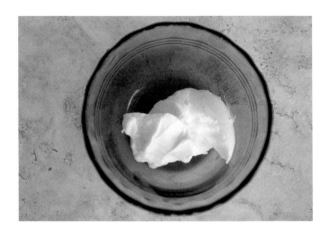

*Precautions:* Water in any product does mean it can be susceptible to mold and fungus (which can start growing within 48 hours!); therefore, a preservative will always be necessary for a decent shelf life. Shelf-stable lotions and creams can last safely for a year. (If I have ordered a larger quantity of lotion or cream, I take out what I need, place it in an essential oil–safe glass or PET plastic container, and store the rest in the refrigerator to prolong its shelf life, with plastic wrap touching the top of the substance and any air bubbles smoothed down to eliminate any unwanted oxygen exchange.)

summer months, as they can feel a bit cooling in winter due to the water content in the base. As a massage therapist, I would sometimes switch to a thicker cream and add gentle warming essential oils in winter.

Lotions have a "looser" feel to them, are emollient (skin softening), and can be rubbed into the skin fairly easily without any heavy residue. Creams are a bit thicker and generally stay on the skin a tad longer. This is helpful if you need to rub an area for a while, such as a sore muscle, or if the skin seems dry; in such situations, the extra hydration of a cream would be preferable over a lotion. Lotions are usually pumpable, whereas creams are generally too thick to go through the pumping mechanism. (Although larger pumps that can handle a thick cream, manufactured for massage therapists, are available for general consumers, the container usually holds much more than most people would use for private home use.)

**Salves** are thicker than creams and more solid than oils, yet act similarly to oils when applied to the skin. Salves are a blend of beeswax, herbal oils, and essential oils, and have a substantial, slick feel. They are wonderful to make and I include a basic recipe to try for yourself. Use for sore muscles and superdry skin applications, and for chest and back rubs during cold and flu season. Salves are intended for smaller areas of the body, whereas oils, lotions, and creams can be used all over the body.

*Precautions:* Do not use salves on weepy skin conditions, acne, infections, burns, poison ivy, pimples, boils, fresh sunburn, or bacterial skin infections.

**Gels** combine aloe vera and hydrosols. Distilled water can be used, but creating gels is the perfect time to experiment with the joy of hydrosols. Be aware that there are two types of aloe vera: gel and

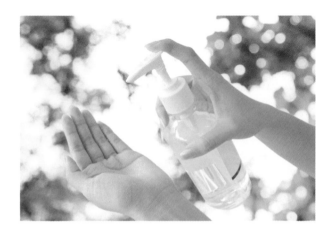

guishing "whole leaf" and "inner fillet." The layer between the outside skin and the inner fillet contains a yellow sap that is counterproductive to healing and can be toxic in large doses. Madeleine Kerkhof-Knapp Hayes, author of *Complementary Nursing in End of Life Care* and an international leader in palliative care with essential oils, suggests using the "inner fillet" only.

**Water:** If water is used for any essential applications, such as diffusers or room spritzers, go with filtered and/or distilled. In a pinch, tap water can be used, but keep in mind that it contains chemical agents, such as chlorine. Distilled water is also recommended for cleaning the face and neck area, according to acupuncturist and herbalist Sarah Crow. Please read the section on dispersants (pages 258–59) for information about the safe distribution of water and essential oils together.

**Hydrosols**, also called hydrolats or flower waters, can be substituted for water in all essential oil applications that require water (including facial washes and diffusers).

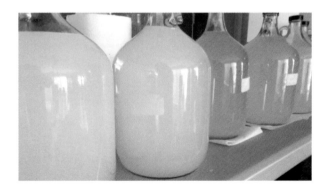

juice. What you want is the gel, which is thicker and slippery, perfect to spread or spray on the skin.

Gels have a unique attribute of being water heavy. When essential oils are combined with gels and applied to the skin, the oils are going to separate out and gravitate toward the natural oils in the skin and away from the gel base, increasing the absorption of the essential oils.

Gel is the most appropriate carrier for treatment of fungal applications and sunburns, and can be used for wounds (if the wound is not weeping) and skin care. Weepy skin conditions, acne, infections, burns, poison ivy, pimples, boils, fresh sunburn, or bacterial skin infections are best suited for cooling water-based remedies, using gels, poultices, or compresses (oil bases could exacerbate these conditions). You can also create an aloe vera gel spritzer that is more fluid, to use as a great first-aid treatment for delicate wounds where any rubbing might not be desired.

*Precaution:* Aloe vera is sometimes sold distin-

*Precautions:* Hydrosols have a shelf life and must be used within a reasonable amount of time. I once had two perfectly good, unopened hydrosols go bad purely because they sat in my refrigerator for too long. Hydrosols should not be used for any skin applications if they bloom (i.e., they look milky, discolored, or develop free-floating threads, meaning bacteria are beginning to grow). In amber or blue bottles, it can be hard to tell whether a hydrosol is going bad; sometimes an off scent will give it away. If in doubt, do not use. Instead, add it to your plants outside.

**Soaps** used for carrier purposes are best if mild, unscented, and liquid. Essential oils added for personal and kitchen use can then be chosen based on scent and/or therapeutics, depending on your intention. Castile soap is a botanical olive oil and sodium hydroxide–based formula safe for all ages, but check whether your added essential oils are child safe: Use unscented soaps (no essential oils added) for all children under 6 months of age and only extremely lightly scented for children over 6 months of age. (For babies 6 months and older, use 0.5% dilution; for 2 years old, 1% is plenty for young bodies as they do not need daily exposure to essential oils). For older kids and adults, unscented liquid hand soaps are very easy to prepare; use fun, uplifting, or grounding oils as desired. (Hard soaps are not covered in this book; they require a fixed oil base that involves a bit more understanding of chemistry to not be harsh on the skin and not too soft to hold their shape.) Unscented emulsified liquid body wash, shampoo,

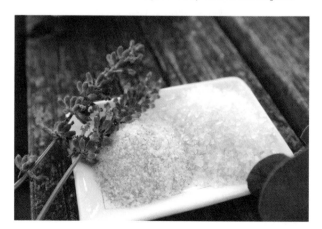

and bubble bath can also be used as a base for dispersing essential oils in a bath without leaving a slick residue on the tub.

**Salts**, usually called bath salts, can be used as foot or hand soaks, or for sitz baths as well as tub baths. Use Epsom salts, Himalayan pink salt, Dead Sea salt, sea salt, or a combination. Changing up the salts gives different textures and colors, as well as slightly different ecological therapeutics depending on where the salts were harvested. Salts are water loving and essential oils are oil loving, so infusing essential oils into dry salts with a little oil (e.g., a teaspoon of jojoba) creates a chemical bond that makes the essential oils safer to use when added to water. However, the added carrier may make the tub slick, so be mindful. See pages 104 and 107 for how to use salts wisely.

## Basic Carrier and Herbal Infused Oils

**Carrier oils:** The following eight oils will get you started. There are many more that have different feels, uses, and scents. Feel free to mix and play with different carriers according to your needs.

- Coconut oil
- Jojoba
- Sesame oil
- Sweet almond oil

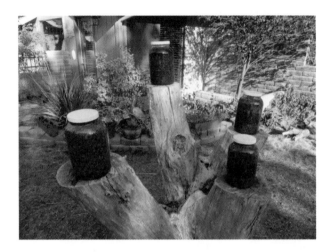

- Apricot kernel oil
- Rosehip seed oil
- Grapeseed oil
- Foraha (tamanu) oil

**Herbal infused oils:** The following are great starter herbal oils to enhance your carrier base as well as give you options for salve making. Herbal oils are usually sold in smaller quantities and are more expensive than other carrier base oils, so it is often used in collaboration with other carriers.

- Arnica
- St. John's wort
- Helichrysum
- Calendula

# WHICH OIL FOR WHICH USE?

Here is a quick list of possible carriers for your essential oil blends. Although some are not covered in this book, I felt it was important for you to begin to expand your awareness of the many options! *Caution:* Make sure you read their profile thoroughly and check with the recipient for any potential allergies before using.

- Dry skin: olive oil, avocado, macadamia, almond, sesame, jojoba, apricot kernel, borage, evening primrose, carrot seed, rosehip seed, foraha/tamanu, shea butter
- Very dry skin: tamanu, shea oil or butter, macadamia
- Normal skin: apricot kernel, almond, argan, avocado, baobab, coconut, jojoba, carrot seed, safflower
- Oily skin: jojoba, rosehip seed, grapeseed, borage, cranberry seed, almond, hazelnut, apricot kernel, mango butter, foraha/tamanu (small amounts to prevent scarring), cucumber, evening primrose, watermelon seed
- Mature/antiaging oils: avocado, argan, marula, macadamia nut, jojoba, moringa, pomegranate seed, rosehip seed, sea buckthorn, black currant
- Massage oils: almond, apricot kernel, avocado, safflower, coconut, jojoba, olive, macadamia, sesame, shea oil, sunflower (heavy butters and creams, such as shea, cocoa, or mango, need to be combined with lighter oils)
- Hair-nutritive carriers: for hair loss: jojoba, borage, evening primrose; for scalp nourishment: coconut, sesame, jojoba
- Children: jojoba; if no nut allergies: baobab, foraha/tamanu (for dry skin), almond, apricot kernel, coconut

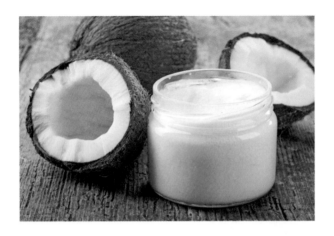

## COCONUT OIL

Grown in tropical climates, coconut (*Cocos nucifera*) is used for its edible meat (fresh and dried); and its water (the liquid inside young coconuts), for drinking. Coconut cream is the first press of fresh mature coconut meat shavings; coconut milk is the second press. Coconut oil is extracted centrifugally from the milk and fresh meat (not the dried meat, called copra), without the use of solvents (Parker 2014).

Coconut oil is a beautiful white solid at temperatures below 76°F and in cold environments, but will begin to melt into a liquid if warmer than 76°F. Thus, solid coconut oil will melt easily when in contact with the heat of your hand and body. True virgin coconut oil possesses the wonderfully sweet aroma known only to coconut. If it has been processed, the scent is reduced or eliminated. Good coconut oil should smell like coconuts.

Fractionated coconut oil (FCO) is coconut oil that has gone through a separation process that produces a clear, rather than white, oil that will not go solid at 76°F. It is often used by massage therapists and for blends that need to remain in a suspended state without the risk of becoming solid. Aromatherapist and massage therapist Rose Chard does not recommend FCO if the blend is intended for a symbiotic relationship with the person and the essential oils. For its full therapeutic benefits, she urges using the oil as nature made it with its complete components and aroma.

*Precautions:* Anyone who has sensitivities or allergies to nuts are encouraged to do a little skin test to ascertain whether coconut sensitivities or allergies apply to the oil as well. Another option is to do a sniff test. (This is *not* a scientific evaluation, but can be an early indicator. The body can sometimes let you know if something is a match or not—this is not the same as asking whether the person likes the scent.) Hold the oil close to the face and sniff the oil. If any physical sensations, tingling, or odd feelings occur, it might be best to skip this oil. If in doubt, choose another oil. If using, I suggest dilution rather than full strength.

Characteristics:
- Aromatic, distinctive coconut odor
- Contains beneficial fatty acids, such as lauric acid (found in tropical oils)
- Compatible with all skin types
- Good for sensitive skin
- Nongreasy
- Antifungal, antimicrobial, antibacterial
- Protects skin from harsh sun; allows vitamin D to be processed without clogging pores, limits

damage from the sun (not to be confused with sunscreen)
- Soothes rashes and inflamed skin
- Dilutes adverse skin reactions to essential oils
- Helps prevent stretch marks
- Hydrating (although sensitive skin may find it too drying if used undiluted)
- Hair tonic, used to massage into the scalp
- Skin tonic, used to soften
- Cleanser, used to clean skin
- In Ayurveda, considered a "cooling" oil for the body; best used for heat-related conditions, to cool them down (also good in the summer)
- Stable shelf life
- Can be used at 100% or blended

## JOJOBA

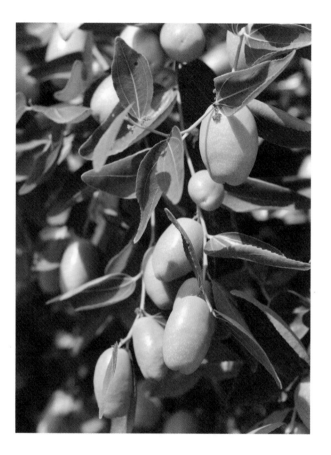

Jojoba (*Simmondsia chinensis*) is native to desert areas of the southwestern United States and northern Mexico. Historically, jojoba (pronounced *ho-HO-ba*) has been used in its region to soothe abrasions, bruises, and burns, and for hair care. A liquid wax ester, it looks like and acts an oil, but without the greasy feel; however, it can solidify like a wax if it gets cold.

Botanically the wax protects the plant against water loss, maintaining a barrier while allowing its stomata to breathe (see page 48); jojoba acts similarly when applied to skin. This makes it an ideal carrier for maintaining moisture, protecting and harmonizing the skin's natural sebum. It is a wonderfully neutral carrier oil, able to blend well with synergies and good for all skin types, whether used alone or in a blend with other carriers. Jojoba can be more expensive than some other carriers, but is worth having some on hand due to its versatility.

Sharon Parker reminds us that jojoba was first brought onto the market in the 1970s as a substitute for sperm whale oil.

Characteristics:

- No aroma; easily showcases essential oil scents
- Contains fatty acids, proteins, vitamin E, and minerals
- Light texture, nongreasy
- Penetrates into the skin easily, while providing a layer of protection on the surface
- Does not clog pores
- Aids acne, eczema, and psoriasis
- Reduces wrinkles
- Balances the natural pH balance of skin
- Can be used in facial preparations at 10 to 20%
- Promotes nail health
- Anti-inflammatory
- Good for oily or combination skin (but can be used by all skin types)
- Lessens dry scalp and dandruff when used in hair care and scalp massage
- Prevents or reduces stretch marks
- Can be used as a cleanser for the face
- Stable shelf life, long lasting
- Can be used at 100% or blended

## SESAME OIL

The words "Open sesame!" were my first introduction as a child to this seed. The joke in the story "Ali Baba and the Forty Thieves" is that Ali Baba's brothers cannot remember the exact words and confuse it with other grains, thus getting trapped in a cave. While the phrase has its first documentation from Antoine Galland's eighteenth-century *Les Mille et une nuits* (The Thousand and One Nights), even

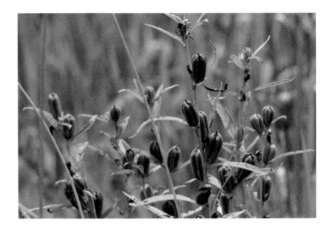

that quotation still does not go back as far as the history of the sesame.

Sesame (*Sesamum indicum*) is one of the oldest seed crops, with more than 5,000 years of cultivation and ancient documentation in India. Ayurveda, Egyptian, and Chinese history all noted sesame's use for food and medicines. Greeks and Romans ate the seeds. Ghilean Prance and Mark Nesbitt's *The Cultural History of Plants* shares, "The first century AD book, *Periplus of the Erythraean Sea*, describes trade in sesame oil from India to the Red Sea ports in exchange for frankincense."

As an oil, sesame contains two of the most powerful antioxidants: sesamolin and sesamin. The warming nature often associated with Ayurveda's use of sesame oil hints of the plant's surviving extreme weather conditions, such as drought, which assists the oil's ability to protect from sun damage. This also makes sesame resistant to oxidization. Sesame is best used as an unrefined source, rather than the toasted sesame oil often used in Asian cuisine.

*Precautions:* Anyone who has sensitivities or allergies to sesame or seeds is encouraged to do a little skin test to ascertain whether these sensitivities or allergies apply to sesame oil as well. Optionally, do a sniff test. If in doubt, choose another oil.

Characteristics:
- Aromatic, nutty, deep scent, heavy, distinctive
- Contains vitamins, minerals, proteins, lecithin (helps the brain and nerves, and removes fats and cholesterol from blood), amino acids, and more
- Helps protect skin from sun damage (not to be confused with sunscreen)
- Moisturizing
- Warming; good for cold weather/environments, cold feelings, or cold body
- Penetrates into skin, goes to deeper layers
- Anti-inflammatory, antioxidant, antibacterial
- Aids healing of capillaries in deep skin layers
- Harmonizes skin sebum; good for acne and dry scalp and skin
- Shelf stable; resistant to oxidation
- Can be used at 100% or blended

## SWEET ALMOND OIL

Thought to have originated in western Asia or the Mediterranean, sweet almond (*Prunus amygdalis* var. *dulcis*, sometimes classified as *Amygdalis communis*), comes from the Rosaceae family (the same

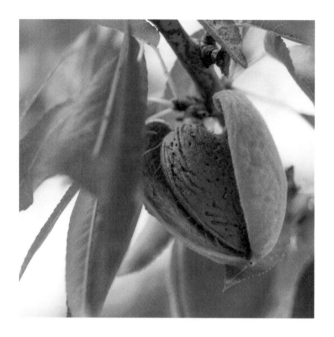

family as rose). Like its cousins the plum, peach, and apricot, almond trees produce stone fruits, called drupes, fruit that contain a pit. What the general public calls a nut is actually a kernel found inside the pit of the fruit; the oil is pressed from the kernel.

*Precautions:* Anyone who has sensitivities or allergies to almonds is encouraged to do a little skin test to ascertain whether these sensitivities or allergies apply to almond oil as well. Optionally, do a sniff test. If in doubt, choose another oil.

Characteristics:
- Aromatic, low, nearly odorless
- Contains fatty acids, trace minerals, oleic acid, and vitamin E

- Considered a light-textured oil
- Assists with collagen maintenance
- Retains moisture and prevents water loss on the skin
- Anti-inflammatory
- Mild and gentle; can be used with children
- Can be used in face oil preparations
- Helps dislodge dirt and blackheads
- Improves skin barrier protective layer
- Benefits dry skin, including eczema and relieves itching due to dryness
- Helps with rashes
- Used for hair and scalp health
- Good base for massage, emollient (glides on skin)
- Best stored in the refrigerator; considered moderately stable with a shelf life of 6 to 12 months
- Can be used at 100% or blended

## APRICOT KERNEL OIL

Apricot (*Prunus armeniaca*) comes from the same family, Rosaceae, as sweet almond oil. Apricot as a fruit-bearing tree is believed to have been domesticated in China 3,000 years ago. Its fruit was known as the "precious one" by Romans.

The apricot kernels are pressed for their naturally nourishing oil that has a light almondlike fragrance. The texture is similar to that of almond oil, but with a slightly softer touch on the skin due to its slightly higher component of linoleic acid. Linoleic acid is important in maintaining a good barrier on the skin, protecting it from bacteria while keeping in moisture. Apricot kernel oil is a lovely choice for lightly scenting your base blend with a natural nutritive oil.

*Precautions:* Anyone who has sensitivities or allergies to tree nuts is encouraged to do a little skin test to ascertain whether these sensitivities or allergies apply to apricot oil as well. Optionally, do a sniff test. If in doubt, choose another oil.

Characteristics:
- Aromatic, light almond scent
- Contains GLA, oleic acid, and vitamins A and E
- Emollient (slides on the skin)
- Anti-inflammatory
- Good for face preparations and body care
- Benefits dry or sensitive skin
- Antiaging; excellent for mature or aging skin
- Antioxidant
- Moderately stable; lasts 6 to 12 months; best kept in the refrigerator
- Can be used at 100%, but is usually used at a 10 to 50% ratio to other base oils

## ROSEHIP SEED OIL

Rosehip (*Rosa rubiginosa*) comes from the hips of the fruit left behind after rose petals have been released by the plant. This wild rose grows around the world, although originally this oil came from Europe and South Africa, and most notably the wild Chilean rose. Rosehip seed oil contains vitamins C and E as well as many other skin-healing properties.

Rosehip seed oil, sometimes referred to as rose-

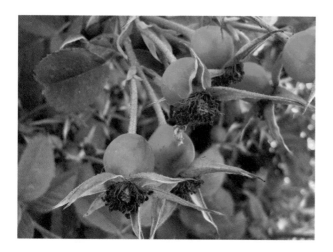

- Absorbs and penetrates skin quickly
- Protects skin barrier
- Cellular regenerator and rejuvenator
- Helps reduce scars and heal burns
- Promotes collagen formation
- Use for mature or prematurely aging skin
- Benefits dry skin
- Use as facial oil in 10 to 20% dilution
- Helps skin damaged by sun or UV exposure, as well as dark spots and uneven pigmentation
- Must be used in a short period of time, stored in a refrigerator
- Can be used as high as 100% for very dry skin; recommended in smaller proportions of 10 to 20% in a blend

hip oil (in Europe, it is sold as muscat, also known as rosa mosquet), is widely revered for its antiaging, hydrating, astringent, scar-reducing, and cellular rejuvenation qualities. It is best used in a blend with other oils at a 10 to 20% dilution. While this oil assists with recovery from acne and does not clog pores, if the skin is acne prone and diet and underlying attributors have not been addressed, it may aggravate the condition. However, if the skin tone is extremely dry, the proportion can be increased to as high as 100% for localized treatment.

This delicate oil should be used in a fairly short time, refrigerated for storage. It would be wise to date the bottle upon purchase, so you can watch the calendar and avoid oxidation.

Characteristics:
- Aromatic, light, pleasant aroma
- Contains numerous fatty acids and vitamins A, C, and E

## GRAPESEED OIL

Grapes (*Vitis vinifera*) are used for wines, grape juice, raisins, table grapes, and both cooking and carrier oils. Although grapes with seeds are no longer com-

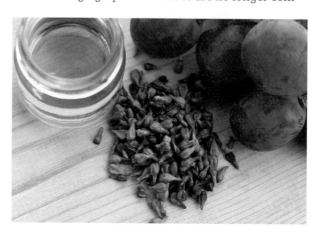

mon in grocery stores, the value of their seed has risen in holistic uses. The common grape, sometimes referred to as the European grape, is a climbing vine native to central Europe, but other species are found in southwestern Asia, the Mediterranean, and even in the United States. Grapes like to be in sun-warmed areas and to be planted in a north–south direction, rather than east–west.

Grapes are technically considered berries. The oil, extracted from the seeds inside the berry, contains a variety of skin-rejuvenating and -repairing properties, including strengthening collagen and maintaining elastin. It emulsifies well (can be mixed with other ingredients); however, its shelf stability is considered moderate and so it should be kept in a cool, dark place.

*Precautions:* if you are allergic to grapes, you may want to avoid this oil. Reactions include headache, dizziness, nausea, elevated blood pressure, and itchy or unusually dry scalp. According to the University of Maryland Medical Center Integrated Wellness website, use should be limited to no more than 12 weeks.

Characteristics:
- Aromatic, light, mild
- Often combined with other oils for massage blends
- Contains fatty acids, such as linoleic acid (light but penetrates skin well) and vitamin E
- Rejuvenates, smooths, and tones skin
- Protects against sun damage and UV rays (not to be confused with sunscreen)

- Moisturizes dry skin
- Benefits eczema and dermatitis
- Can be used in acne blends
- A nice addition to muscle, joint, or trauma support blends
- Antioxidant, anti-inflammatory, analgesic, antioxidant
- Helps heal wounds and may reduce swelling from injuries
- Aids circulation and capillary repair
- Shelf stability is moderate, 6 to 12 months, best stored in a cool, dark place
- Can be used up to 100% or blended in small dilutions with other carrier oils

## FORAHA (TAMANU) OIL

*Calophyllum inophyllum*, Greek for "beautiful leaf," is known by many names, depending on the island or region to which you are referring, thus the Latin binomial is helpful when referring for specific

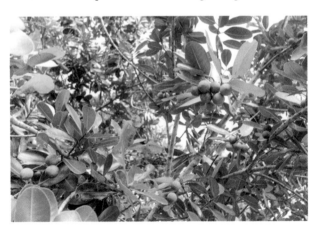

needs or communications. This thick, aromatic oil is called foraha (*for-AH-ha*) in Madagascar and tamanu (*TAH-mah-noo*) in Polynesia (its other names around the Pacific region include faraha, kamanu, kamani, fetau, and dilo oil). This tropical tree is heavy in nutrients, scent, color, and uses. The oil is obtained from the tree nut, but only after it has dried, as fresh nuts produce no oil. The process takes about 8 weeks. By the end of the drying time, a third of the nut's weight is oil, making it a high-yield product easily obtained by expeller pressing. The oil is deep green and its scent is strong and nutty.

Foraha's benefits are numerous, but its heavy scent is sometimes avoided when making softer-scented blends. However, this oil is often utilized by aromatherapists for its powerful therapeutics. It contains a unique-to-the-tree chemical compound, calophyllolide, a strong anti-inflammatory agent. When combined with rosehip seed oil, greatly assists wound healing and scar formation along with adhesions, and even deep keloid scars have been softened.

*Precautions:* Anyone who has sensitivities or allergies to tree nuts are encouraged to do a little skin test to ascertain whether foraha sensitivities or allergies apply to the oil as well. Optionally, do a sniff test. If in doubt, choose another oil. If there are no indications, I suggest dilution rather than full strength.

Characteristics:
- Aromatic, heavily aromatic, nutty
- Deeply penetrating
- Contains fatty acids, oleic acid, linoleic acid, palmitic acid, stearic acid, and calophyllolide
- Benefits dry skin, very dry, and damaged skin
- Regenerates skin
- Helps heal wounds and burns
- Use for cuts, scrapes, and insect bites and stings
- Reduces pain attributed to joint, arthritis, neuralgia, rheumatism, and sciatica
- Good as a base oil in blends for shingles
- Promotes scar reduction associated with acne and/or skin trauma
- Antioxidant, anti-inflammatory, antimicrobial, antibacterial, analgesic
- Prevents infections
- Use in blends for eczema, psoriasis, and stretch marks
- Helps heal blisters, cold sores, and herpes sores
- Stable, shelf life up to 2 years if stored in a refrigerator; the oil will solidify when cold, so take out 30 minutes prior to use
- Can be used at 100%, but due to its strong aroma, it is more commonly used as 15 to 20% of an overall blend

# Herbal Carrier Oils

### ARNICA HERBAL OIL

Arnica (*Arnica montana*), which grows wild in mountain areas in the northern United States and many places throughout Europe, has a long history

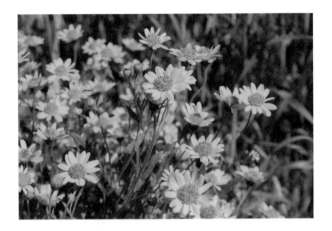

of assisting the body with trauma repair. It expedites healing by increasing circulation to the localized area, bringing in new blood, fresh oxygen, nutrients, and white blood cells to help repair and clean up any pooled blood, such as bruises. By reducing swelling and increasing circulatory flow after surgery or physical trauma, arnica often reduces pain, in turn reducing the need for pain medications. Arnica herbal oil is often made by soaking the flowers in olive oil for 3 to 4 weeks before straining.

Characteristics:
- Highest-rated oil for soft tissue trauma, as well as benefits bumps and hematomas due to trauma
- Reduces pain
- Anti-inflammatory
- Reduces bruising and swelling
- Helps with shock
- Good for sprains and joint and muscle aches

## ST. JOHN'S WORT HERBAL OIL

St. John's wort (*Hypericum perforatum*) is known as hypericum (pronounced *hi-PEH-rih-come*) in homeopathy. This versatile oil comes from a yellow blossoming herb with a rhizome base. Although many consider it a weed, as it can be invasive, I have found it to be quite beautiful at my local botanical gardens. It is native to Europe and Asia, but has spread worldwide, and is fond of temperate conditions. It blooms in the summer, usually by June 24, which is the feast day of St. John the Baptist, thus its name. The herbal oil must be made from fresh flowers, so harvesting and cultivating is done only once a year. Historically, the plant has been used as an herb in many cultures, in homeopathy, and in Traditional Chinese Medicine to move stuck liver qi that may be producing depression and blocking creative flow. Commonly infused in an olive oil base.

*Precautions:* If you are sensitive to St. John's wort, do not use this oil. Sensitivities can include

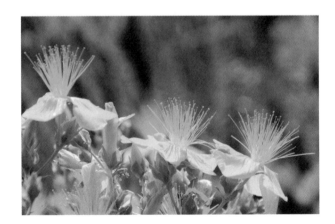

vivid dreams, anxiousness, confusion, digestive upset, headache, restlessness, or sedation. Do not use if you are taking blood thinners, you have been diagnosed with depression, or during pregnancy or breastfeeding. Photosensitive properties are present in orally taken St. John's wort. Although they are not believed to be present in oils used externally (Tisserand and Young 2014), to be safe, use this herbal oil under clothing or at night, and avoid direct sunlight or UV exposure. If in doubt, consult your physician or certified or clinical aromatherapist. Store in the refrigerator when not in use, and do not use if oxidized or rancid smelling.

Characteristics:
- Aromatic with heavy texture
- Contains vitamins A, B1, B2, B6, B6, and D as well as linoleic acid
- Relieves depression and mood swings
- Soothes dry skin, but can be used for all skin types
- Reduces PMS symptoms and menopausal mood swings
- Calms the nervous system
- Eases pain and discomfort
- Helps support liver function
- Provides anti-inflammatory benefits to burns, scrapes, scars, and soft tissues
- Often combined with arnica or calendula to support trauma healing, reduce pain
- Lessens redness or soreness in overworked and tense muscles

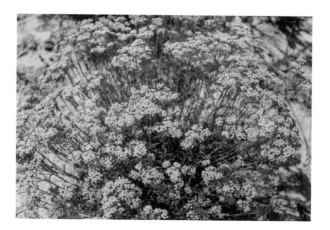

## HELICHRYSUM HERBAL OIL

Helichrysum (*Helichrysum italicum*), pronounced *hel-ih-KRY-sum* ("sun" and "gold"), is one of the top skin-support herbal infused oils and is a wonderful addition to soothing skin blends (see also page 000 to read about helichrysum essential oil). The grayish green foliage is topped with bright yellow flowers, hence the name. I use this oil whenever I want to support any kind of proper skin harmony, from a bump or a bruise to easing dry skin. Commonly infused in an olive oil base.

Characteristics:
- Rejuvenates skin
- Repairs trauma
- Provides cellular support for proper functioning
- Antibacterial, antifungal, anti-inflammatory
- Benefits dry skin
- Works on the deep layers of the skin
- Soothes physical and emotional scars

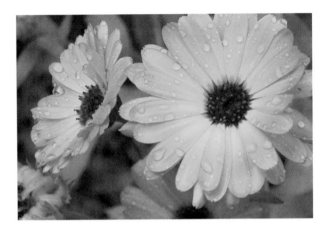

- Good for eczema, psoriasis, and skin ulcers
- Anti-inflammatory and antispasmodic
- Promotes healing of wounds or damaged tissues
- Provides postsurgical skin repair
- Helps skin irritations and rashes, such as diaper rash
- Soothes insect bites and burns
- Can be used 100% or in blends with other oils; recommended blend dilution is 15 to 25%

## Preservatives, Antioxidants, Emulsifiers, and Dispersants

The only way to get products to last longer on the shelf of your bathroom or vanity is to add a *preservative*, to keep them free of fungus and bacterial growth. All water-based products need a preservative if you plan on making more than a few days' worth. Knowing which preservative you are choosing is right for your product involves knowing pH levels and a bit of chemistry to ensure broad-spectrum preservation, which is beyond the scope of this book. If a beginner, you can start with a commercially made unscented lotion or cream as a means to avoid adding a preservative yourself, since they are designed to have a preserved shelf life of about one year. Heed precautions and dilutions according to safe practices as you add your essential oils. *Carrier oils alone do not need preservatives*, unless a water agent is added to them. Most carriers have a shelf life of about one year, some longer, if properly stored.

- Supports proper immune function
- Can be used 100% or in a blend

## CALENDULA HERBAL OIL

Calendula (*Calendula officinalis*) is another herb used across the board as a plant, homeopathically, medicinally, and infused in olive oil as an herbal carrier oil. Calendula has been used for skin care in everything from baby products to lotions and creams, and can be found in body butters and oils, such as this carrier oil. It has a reputation for reaching the deeper layers of the body, which is helpful for wound healing as well as for calming inflammation. Calendula herbal oil can be used for all ages. It is often infused with an olive oil base.

Characteristics:
- Contains vitamins, A, E, proteins, lecithin, amino acids, and antioxidants
- Aromatic
- Rejuvenates and hydrates skin

Note: Lotions and creams can hold a bit of essential oil; however, adding too many ingredients can alter the ratio of the lotion, hence changing its chemistry.

Vitamin E and rosemary extracts, once thought to be natural preservatives, are in fact antioxidants. *Antioxidants* delay the oxidation. Adding a few drops to a blend or synergy, lotion, or cream, still does not prevent bacteria or fungi from growing. Bacteria can begin to grow with a day or two. For these reasons, the recipes in this book are designed to be simple and do not require preservation, although you can have the added benefit of a drop or two of vitamin E to your topical blends. Susan M. Parker suggests the following carrier oils as helpers in maintaining longer shelf lives due to molecular stability: meadowfoam, marula, moringa, and baobab, as well as vitamin E (2014).

The best antioxidant is not vitamin E from your grocery store. The easiest for a home user to purchase is a commercial vitamin E product, such as Tocobiol® SF. Rosemary Antioxidant $CO_2$ is also available and has been shown to out-perform vitamin E as an excellent antioxidant. In both cases, they will need to be ordered as they not normally found in local stores.

Generally speaking, for home use, keep your blends as clean as possible, make small batches, and use as often as appropriate. Do not allow water to enter your product (e.g., humidity from the hot shower or reaching in with wet hands). Toss the blend if the color shifts or the scent acquires rancid notes. Bacteria can grow before you see/smell it (as quickly as 48 hours in water-based products!).

*Emulsifiers* and *dispersants* are different from preservatives. To emulsify means to add two compounds to each other in a way that they mix, creating a new item, allowing the two original ingredients to stay suspended and not separate. Lotion is an example of mixing oil and water in a way that it changes because it has been emulsified. Using emulsifiers and dispersants can help distribute essential oils to combine in a water base easily; for instance, in a bath, bug repellent, or room-freshening spray.

A common and easy-to-use dispersant is Solubol, in a dilution ratio of 1:4 dispersant to essential oils (e.g., add 3 drops Solubol to every 12 drops of essential oil). Add to room spray mists (not diffusers), linen sprays, bath salts, or milk bath creations to further disperse them safely in water. Other dispersants (for baths) are liquid oil-based soaps (Castile), body wash, or shampoos. Full-fat milk and cream, bath agents since antiquity, may or may not disperse the oils as well as an already emulsified agent. To be safe, choose oils that have low dermal sensitive potentials.

Alcohol used as a dispersant can be self-preserving as well as good for suspending essential oils for room-spray mists and linen sprays (but may be too drying for topical application). (Use 190 proof alcohol to fill the container at least a quarter full; fill the rest of the way with distilled water—not tap water.) Using 100% alcohol can irritate the lungs if sprayed frequently, but does work well as a dispersant.

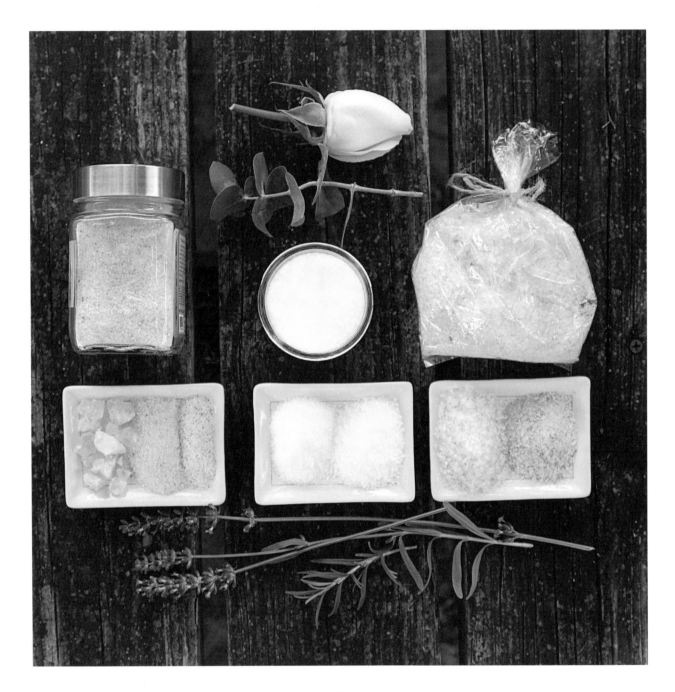

# CHAPTER 17

# Recies

**Following a recipe leads you down the path of creative, meaningful, and thoughtful connections to the essential oils.** However, blending essential oils as a general rule usually has personal needs in mind.

I suggest you play with these remedies to strengthen your observation of how they smell, work, and feel, and how *you* feel. If you do not have one of the ingredients, but have something similar; for instance, you do not have sweet orange, but you have tangerine, by all means substitute tangerine (make sure you know the contraindications of each oil before substituting)! You may find it helpful to record your thoughts and observations while you experiment with these gifts from nature. Enjoy!

A few quick notes to help you with your recipes.

- *Personal inhalers* vary from holding 15 to 30 drops of essential oils. I have worked with both. If you overload a wick designed to only hold 15 drops, it will leak all over (not good to waste your essential oils this way, nor will you like the mess it makes in a travel bag or purse). Check your supplier for the suggested number of drops for that wick or supply your own by using a clean, organic cotton ball you roll into a wick. You can add a drop or two of jojoba to the wick; this may keep some of the essential oils from drying out quickly. Inhalers can last a couple of months.

- *Diffusers* can range in how much water they hold, but average with a run time of 3 hours on $1/3$ cup of water. Adding 3 to 5 drops of essential oils will be plenty. If is recommended to run diffusers intermittently for 30 minutes, then leave off for at least an hour or two. Children need less exposure time, running only 15 to 30 minutes, then turning off. Set a timer to remind you to turn the diffuser off (I use my oven timer when I am at home). At the end of the day, discard the unused water and wipe dry with a clean cloth or paper towel to keep bacteria growth at bay.

- *Commercially available unscented creams and lotions* have a shelf life averaging about a year, but if they start to look or smell bad, discard immediately.
- *Label* with date, product name, and list of ingredients.

# MIND AND HEART
## Memory and Study

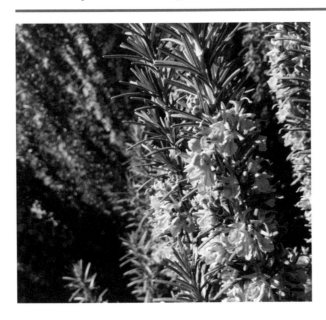

This combination is wonderful while preparing for a presentation, studying, and for those who are having a hard time remembering details. Great for teens through age 100+ (see page 134 for cineole safety).

**Inhaler:**

2 drops rosemary ct. verbenone

3 drops rosemary ct. cineole

2 drops ginger

5 drops mandarin or sweet orange

**Room diffuser:**

1 drop rosemary ct. verbenone

1 drop rosemary ct. cineole

1 drop ginger

2 drops mandarin or sweet orange

# Peaceful Blend

**Add to a personal inhaler:**

5 drops sandalwood

5 drops frankincense

5 drops cedarwood

1 to 2 drops marjoram *or* 1 to 2 drops silver fir or pine (optional)

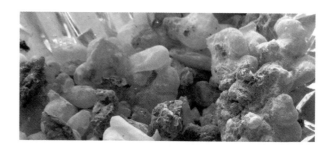

# Frustration Soother

For when times are rough on the emotional heart with a lot of anger and frustration. Best if used in a diffuser or personal inhaler. You can, however, create a wonderful lotion or carrier oil base as part of your daily self-care routine. It is grounding, pacifying to the nervous system and cooling the heat of emotions.

**Inhaler** (*optional: diffuser, reduce drops to 1 drop of each oil, with 2 drops of lavender*)**:**

5 drops palmarosa

1 to 2 drops patchouli or vetiver

1 drop Roman chamomile

6 drops lavender

**Lotion:**

Create the following synergy, then add to 1 ounce of lotion or cream:

6 to 7 drops palmarosa

1 to 2 drops patchouli or vetiver

1 drop Roman chamomile

7 to 8 drops lavender

# BODY
## Cough Soother Room Diffuser (children ages 6+)

3 drops *Eucalyptus globulus (see first note)*

2 drops ginger

1 drop cistus (see note)

*Notes: Substitute rosalina or cedarwood for E. globulus for younger children. Run the diffuser for 15 to 30 minutes, then turn it off for an hour or two.*

*Cistus is a unique aroma and may be a little unusual for some at first, but it is great to add for its ability to aid in opening respiratory airways and to calm the nervous system.*

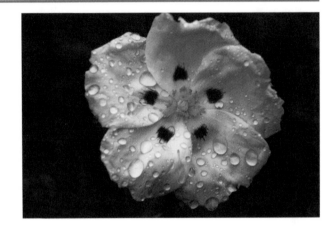

## Lavender Dreams

This is a nice end-of-day lotion for hands, arms, and chest. Apply after a shower or before going to bed.

Mix into 2 ounces of unscented lotion or cream:

25 drops lavender

10 to 15 drops rose geranium

8 to 10 drops palo santo

# Acne Facial Oil

This oil soothes and repairs skin, plus supports emotional calm and well-being.

Combine in a 1-ounce glass bottle with the orifice reducer removed:

2 drops neroli

2 drops Roman chamomile

4 drops patchouli

1 drop frankincense (*Boswellia frereana or B. carteri*)

1 drop dawn-blooming jasmine (optional, this is a very expensive oil!)

40 drops (4 ml) apricot kernel oil (carrier)

20 drops (2 ml) rosehip seed oil (carrier)

Jojoba (carrier) to fill the rest of the way

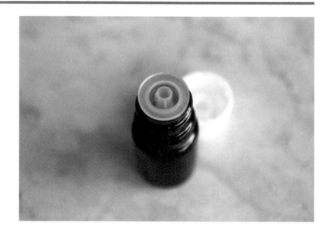

*Notes: Always smell the synergy of essential oils first before adding the carrier oils so that you can identify the fragrance and fragrance intensity. Facial oils should be light and lovely, and in low dilution. Nine drops total will place this at a 1.5% dilution rate, safe for facial application.*

*Replace the orifice reducer and use 1 to 2 drops of the blend, dabbed gently on clean skin, morning and night. Label and date; best stored in the refrigerator due to rosehip's delicate shelf life.*

# Stomach, Skin, and Mind Relaxer

This blend (used externally only) soothes an upset stomach, especially bloating or flatulence after overindulging. The skin will benefit from the smoothing properties and the mind will enjoy the relaxing yet uplifting fragrance, centering the spirit. This is a great oil to rub upon the chest, abdomen, lower back, and upper legs at the end of the day to allow for rest. *Caution:* Do not apply this to skin that may be exposed to UV rays or direct sunlight within 12 to 24 hours of application, due to phototoxic compounds found in lemon and bergamot (this recipe is considered safe levels, but it is best to avoid UV rays). Do not use if pregnant or breastfeeding.

Add the following essential oils to 1 ounce of your choice of carrier oil in an amber or cobalt blue glass bottle:

4 drops lemon

3 drops bergamot (see note)

4 drops palo santo

4 drops patchouli

4 drops sweet fennel

*Note: Using 3 drops of bergamot to 1 ounce of carrier is the maximum for safe photosensitivity levels.*

# Hair Tonic

Encourages growth, sebum harmonization, and is good for hair loss.

Create a synergy of the following essential oils in a 1-ounce amber or cobalt blue bottle:

4 drops cedar

8 drops rosemary ct. verbenone

2 drops peppermint

4 drops lavender

2 drops palmarosa

1. Add a blend of the following oils or use singularly: argan, jojoba, coconut, sesame.

2. Starting with the scalp, apply systematically in a massaging action to cover the whole head, using all of the oil. Let sit for 30 minutes to overnight. (I cover my head with a plastic hair cover and put a light towel on my pillow if doing an overnight application.) Wash the hair by applying shampoo to "dry" hair first, massaging in, and then adding water. Repeat if necessary.

*Helpful hint: use a pipette to apply the oil to the scalp with one hand and massage in with the other!*

# End-of-Day Relaxing Blend

This is deeply relaxing with base notes that sing alongside the warmth of spicy ginger and cooling fennel. Use this at the end of the day or during your meditations. Create the following synergy in a 10 ml roller bottle. *Caution:* Omit the fennel if pregnant or breastfeeding.

2 drops patchouli

2 drops frankincense

2 drops fennel

2 drops ginger

Add your choice of carrier oil and place a very small amount (just a couple of drops) on your chest, wrists, and atop the crown of your head. This makes a nice anointing oil. You may replace the carrier oil with lotion if you would like to make this a nice end-of-day foot lotion. You can also use this synergy alone in a personal inhaler. The scent will begin to change over time bringing out more of the deep patchouli notes.

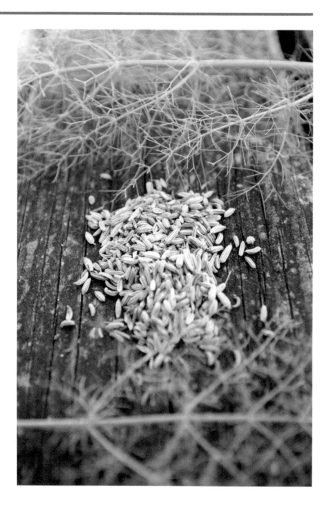

# Basic Salve Recipe

Salves are great for massaging into sore muscles and are often used for assisting respiratory ailments. Caution: All safety protocols apply to essential oils used in personalized blends, especially if intended for reducing pain or for use on children and the elderly. Salves do not contain any water-based ingredients, therefore have a shelf life of 6 to 12 months.

Yields one 2-ounce jar

0.25 ounce of beeswax (measured out on a digital scale)

¼ cup herbal infused oil (St. John's wort, arnica, trauma oil) or your choice of oil (such as jojoba)

30 to 40 drops essential oil synergy for holistic blend (2.5%), or 60 to 90 drops for adult pain blends (5%)

1.  In a clean 2-ounce PET container or amber glass jar, create the essential oil synergy of your choice, allowing the oils to merge together. Cover with lid and set aside.

2.  Fill a deep pot with a sturdy bottom with 2 inches of water. Begin to warm the water on medium high on a stove or hot plate. Place a clean Pyrex 2-cup measuring cup into the pot. Do not allow any water to get *into* the Pyrex cup! You'll have to start over if there is any water mixed in!

3.  Add the beeswax to the Pyrex and allow it to melt slowly (I use beeswax pellets for easier measuring and faster melting). When the beeswax is almost completely melted, add the herbal oil of your choice (the beeswax might temporarily solidify when the oil is added, due to temperature change, but will melt again). Stir with a non-reactive metal spoon or glass stir rod until all is melted.

4.  Have your synergy jar nearby, uncapped. With a towel handy, carefully remove the Pyrex from the water bath (it will be hot!), immediately wiping off all of the hot water on the outside of the container (so no water can drip into the prepared synergy jar, or you'll have to start over!).

5.  Slowly but without hesitation (the beeswax will begin to solidify in the cold air), pour warm oil mixture into your synergy jar. Stir with non-reactive metal spoon or stir stick. Let cool

completely with the container open (unsealed) before using. Label and date. Will last 6 months (up to a year if you store in the fridge).

6. To clean your Pyrex, wipe off as much residue as possible with paper towels, newspaper, or rub it into your skin—this saves your sink and drains. Wash away any remaining residue with plenty of soap.

*A double boiler can be substituted for the Pyrex method.*

Sample synergies:

- *Respiratory:* 16 drops of each rosemary (ct. cineole or ct. verbena), peppermint, and euca-lyptus (*radiata* or *globulos*) (adapted from Jade Shutes). For ages 6 to 12, reduce number of drops by half and avoid using near the head. Do not use on children under 6 due to peppermint.
- *Sprain care:* 10 drops helichrysum, 15 drops lavender, 5 drops black pepper or ginger, 5 drops chamomile, 5 drops marjoram.
- *Sore muscles:* 15 drops juniper berry, 10 drops helichrysum, 10 drops total your choice of pine, fir, or cypress.
- *Skin rejuvenation:* 8 drops helichrysum, 6 drops rose geranium, 15 drops lavender

# BATH

The easiest and safest way to enjoy essential oils in your bath is to dissolve them in an emulsifier base, such as a vegetable-based soap (Castile) or a fat-containing substance, such as cream (full-fat milk), before adding to a bath. As mentioned before, body wash or shampoo can be used to disperse the oil if mixed together before applying to the water. For bath salts, a teaspoon of carrier oil is suggested to disperse the oils safely, but it does tend to make the tub slick with an oily residue. Use the following basic recipes and then change up the essential oils and carriers: Remember to enter the bath first and then add your mixture, to protect sensitive areas from making the first contact.

## Relaxing Bath

1 tablespoon unscented Castile soap, liquid body wash, or shampoo

5 drops lavender

3 drops mandarin

2 drops neroli

Add to a warm, full bath, after you are already sitting in the tub, swishing around the blend to disperse. Enjoy.

## Warming Bath

1 tablespoon unscented Castile soap, liquid body wash, or shampoo

3 drops cardamom

3 drops ginger

8 drops mandarin

Mix well. Once you are in the bath, add mixture to the water, swish to disperse. Enjoy.

# Spirit Soothing Bath Salts

3 drops palo santo

3 drops rose geranium

1 drop Roman chamomile

1 teaspoon coconut, sweet almond, or jojoba carrier oil

1 cup Epsom salts

2 drops Solubol (optional)

Place your choice of essential oils and Solubol, if using, in your choice of carrier mixture in a small glass or ceramic bowl (avoid plastic, reactive metals, and wood). Mix thoroughly. Add the salts and stir to coat evenly. Add to the bath after you are in the water. Swish to dissolve and enjoy. Good for one bath or two foot soaks.

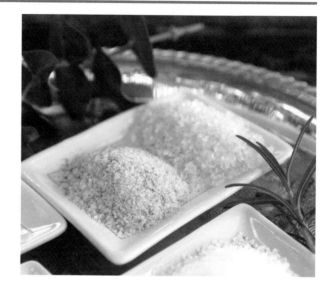

# Hydrosol Bath Time for Children

Hydrosols are wonderful to add to the bath for children instead of essential oils. Add hydrosols to the bath water after the little one is already in the water, to avoid any sensitive skin making first contact. Jade Shutes recommends the following guidelines:

- *Babies 6 months and younger:* 1 teaspoon of hydrosol in an infant bath.
- *Children up to 12 years old:* 1 teaspoon per age of the child, with a maximum of 8 teaspoons. (For

example, 6 years old, maximum 6 teaspoons). Yep, that means all those 9- to 12-year-olds receive a maximum of 8 teaspoons.
- *Adults* may enjoy hydrosols, 1 to 8 ounces max, in a full bath.
- *For a nighttime bath:* add lavender or rose or neroli hydrosol.
- *For a not-feeling-well bath:* try lavender or chamomile hydrosol.
- *For healthy skin:* use helichrysum hydrosol.

# SPIRIT
## Meditation Blend

Create a master synergy with the following essential oils in a 5 ml amber or cobalt blue bottle. From this bottle you can add 1 to 5 drops to your diffuser.

3 to 4 drops ylang-ylang

4 to 5 drops palo santo

4 to 5 drops patchouli

5 to 6 drops sweet orange

1. Once your synergy is complete, place an orifice reducer on the top to help you pour out a single drop at a time. Gently roll the bottle to help the oils combine. Add a drop or two of the total undiluted synergy to a room water diffuser. (Make sure to properly label your synergy!) This is a potent combination; you may find that diffusing for a few minutes may be all you need to set the space.

2. This can also be made into a personal perfume by placing 3 to 5 drops of the undiluted synergy in a 10 ml roller bottle. Top off with jojoba carrier oil. Label properly.

## Desert Sunset

This scent reminds me of the earth's vast desert with the zing of herbaceousness and the far-off scent of desert flowers in the distance. A warm, uplifting synergy to boost self-confidence, reduce anxiety, and create calm focus and a relaxed mind. Good before creative endeavors, sleeping, or quiet meditative moments. Can be made into a master synergy blend.

In a personal inhaler (designed for holding up to 25 drops), combine:

2 drops cistus

2 drops vetiver

6 drops ginger

8 drops palo santo

5 drops patchouli

1 to 2 drops jojoba (carrier; optional)

# Sleep

Add the following to a room water diffuser and run for 30 minutes before going to bed. Turn off the diffuser when you are ready for bed. Alternatively, place drops on a cotton ball and set it on a ceramic or glass plate by your nightstand before you go to bed (do not let the essential oils touch wood or plastic).

2 drops mandarin

2 drops lavender

2 drops neroli

*or*

2 drops bergamot

2 drops lavender

1 drop palo santo

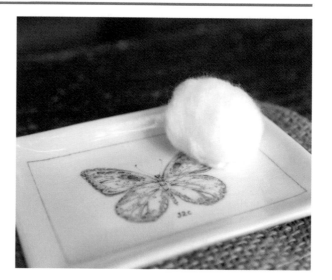

# Confidence

In a personal inhaler, combine:

5 drops mandarin

3 drops neroli

3 drops laurel

3 drops black pepper

Alternatively, use the following blend in a room diffuser:

3 drops mandarin

1 drop neroli

1 drop laurel

1 drop black pepper

# Earth and Sky

This blend is designed to help with letting go, while maintaining groundedness during times of stress. Helps release obstacles and open intuition.

Combine in a personal inhaler (one with a 30-drop cotton wick):

10 drops laurel

5 drops marjoram

4 drops ginger

2 drops palo santo

2 drops patchouli

1 to 2 drops vetiver

1 drop cistus

# Clean Air

This is good for air purification when it feels stagnant, in times of illness, or any time you want to visit the forest from your home or office. Create a master synergy (about 20 drops) in a 5 ml cobalt blue or amber glass bottle; then add 1 to 5 drops to a diffuser. Good for ages 2 and over (you can eliminate *E. radiata* with kids). Run the diffuser for 15 minutes for younger children and up to 30 minutes for adults.

**Master synergy for diffusing:**

4 drops silver fir

4 drops cypress

4 drops cedarwood

4 drops piñon pine

4 drops *Eucalyptus radiata*

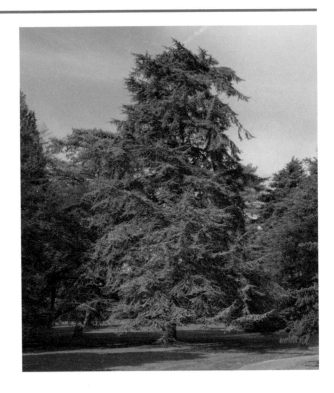

# HOME
## Linen Spray

Combine your choice of oils in a 2-ounce amber or cobalt blue glass bottle with a spray top, then fill ¼ to ½ with 190 proof alcohol (for greatest dispersal); if you use vodka as a substitute, shake before every spray. Top off with distilled water (not tap water). (Use 100% 190 proof alcohol if you do not have distilled water).

**Uplift:**
8 drops lemon
6 drops palmarosa
10 drops sweet orange

**Bedtime:**
12 drops lavender
6 drops sweet orange
4 drops neroli

## Scented Liquid Hand Soap

Add to 4 to 8 ounces of unscented liquid soap (you may adjust for scent, up to 50 drops total, start with these drop measurements then adjust accordingly). Be mindful, as wonderful as these scents are, they are literally going down the drain, as all wash-off products do. Mix well. The scent may change over the course of a couple of days. Best stored in a PET plastic, glass, or glazed ceramic container if on the counter top.

**Rose Geranium Lemon:**
12 drops rose geranium
12 drops lemon

**Lavender Rose:**
15 drops lavender
10 drops rose geranium or palmarosa

**Pine Forest (sweet orange):**
8 drops your choice of white fir, piñon pine, or ponderosa pine
5 drops cypress
5 drops *Eucalyptus radiata*
8 drops sweet orange

**Floral Bliss:**
10 drops ylang-ylang
10 drops patchouli

**Deep Floral:**
5 drops ylang-ylang
5 drops palmarosa
5 drops lavender
5 drops cistus
5 drops patchouli

**Rosemary Eucalyptus:**
12 drops rosemary ct. verbenone
12 drops *Eucalyptus radiata*

## Nighttime Parent Tip

To create a relaxing environment, a few spritz of lavender or Roman chamomile hydrosol can be used in children's rooms or in the air over their bed before they climb in (the bedding should not be dampened). It won't take much, just a few pumps into the air.

## Wake Up

For school-age children who have a hard time waking up in the morning, try diffusing a single drop of lemon or lime essential oil for no more than 15 minutes. (Ages 5 and above.) Diffusing lemon or lime adds additional zip to the senses. Setting a routine at night is the best way to assist an easy morning. Do not diffuse every day, only when needed.

## Bug Bites

Lavender or Roman chamomile can be used in diluted form (1 to 3 drops in a roller bottle filled with a carrier) to help control itching. Undiluted lavender is not recommended.

# Create Your Own Blends

Name of blend: _____   Date: _____

Purpose: _____

Instructions: _____

_____

_____

Essential oils:

_____ drops of _____    _____ drops of _____

_____ drops of _____    _____ drops of _____

Carrier base (oil, lotion, cream, salt, soap, water, etc.): _____

_____

Method of delivery (massage, diffuser, bath, steam, cotton ball, personal inhaler, etc.): _____

_____

Observations: _____

_____

_____

Name of blend: _____  Date: _____

Purpose: _____

Instructions: _____

_____

_____

Essential oils:

_____ drops of _____  _____ drops of _____

_____ drops of _____  _____ drops of _____

Carrier base (oil, lotion, cream, salt, soap, water, etc.): _____

_____

Method of delivery (massage, diffuser, bath, steam, cotton ball, personal inhaler, etc.): _____

_____

Observations: _____

_____

_____

_____

Name of blend: _____ Date: _____

Purpose: _____

Instructions: _____

_____

_____

Essential oils:

_____ drops of _____     _____ drops of _____

_____ drops of _____     _____ drops of _____

Carrier base (oil, lotion, cream, salt, soap, water, etc.): _____

_____

Method of delivery (massage, diffuser, bath, steam, cotton ball, personal inhaler, etc.): _____

_____

Observations: _____

_____

_____

_____

**Absolute:** first phase of solvent extraction, where alcohol is used to create highly aromatic concentrations of the volatile material.

**Adulteration:** when a substance has been altered from its original composition.

**Allelopathy:** when a plant sends a signal to ward off competing plants.

**Analgesic:** relieves pain.

**Antibacterial:** halts and inhibits the growth of bacteria.

**Anticatarrhal:** helps remove excess mucus.

**Anticoagulant:** stops the clotting of blood.

**Antidepressant:** relieves depression.

**Antiemetic:** aids in combating vomiting and nausea.

**Antifungal:** fights fungal infections.

**Anti-infectious:** prevents infections.

**Anti-inflammatory:** reduces inflammation.

**Antimicrobial:** kills microorganisms and/or stops their growth.

**Antipruritic:** soothes the sensation of itching.

**Antirheumatic:** combats rheumatoid arthritis.

**Antiseborrheic:** slows down sebum production.

**Antiseptic:** reduces risk of infections.

**Antispasmodic:** relieves muscle spasms.

**Antitussive:** eases coughing.

**Antiviral:** eradicates viruses.

**Anxiolytic:** diminishes anxiety.

**Aphrodisiac:** enhances romantic or sexual response.

**Aromatherapy:** therapeutic application of essential oils and aromatic plant extracts used to maintain or improve the well-being of an individual physically, mentally, emotionally, and/or spiritually.

**Astringent (syn. styptic):** shrinks or constricts body tissue.

**Bactericide:** eliminates bacteria.

**Balsamic:** soothing.

**Biocompatibility:** when a substance is compatible with another living tissue or system.

**Blend:** when a carrier and one or more essential oils have been mixed together.

**Calmative:** calming.

**Carminative:** diminishes flatulence.

**Cephalic:** aids the head and mind and stimulates thought processes.

**Chemotype:** indicates a chemical type, or variation, of a plant or substance due to a chemical composition change based on environmental conditions.

**Cholagogue:** stimulates the gallbladder in order to increase bile flow.

**Choleretic:** stimulates bile secretion through the liver.

**Cicatrisant:** healing aid by the formation of scar tissue; skin healing.

**CO$_2$ supercritical extraction:** process in which carbon dioxide in a pressurized chamber are used to extract essential oils without heat, steam, or water.

**Common name:** most used name to identify an essential oil.

**Decongestant:** relieves congestion of the respiratory system.

**Deodorant:** eliminates odors.

**Dermal toxicity:** level or potential effect/reaction on the skin from a substance.

**Detoxifier:** eliminates toxins.

**Digestive:** helps the process of digestion.

**Distillation:** process in which steam is used to release the volatile components, using a still.

**Diuretic:** boosts urination.

**Drupe:** thin-skinned fruit surrounding the center-most seed.

**Emmenagogue:** encourages menstruation.

**Emollient:** soothes and softens skin.

**Enfleurage:** extracting the fragrance of a single flower species by using purified animal or vegetable fats.

**Essential oil:** a natural oil extracted by distillation of a single botanical species while retaining its name, odor, and medicinal properties. A volatile vapor extracted from an aromatic plant source. A secondary metabolite.

**External secretory structures:** exterior compartments that hold essential oils on a plant.

**Family:** taxonomic category above genus.

**Febrifuge:** diminishes fever.

**Fungicide:** eliminates fungus.

**Genus (pl. *genera*):** taxonomic category between family and species.

**Hemostatic:** helps stop bleeding.

**Headspace:** area above the top surface of a liquid in a container.

**Hepatic:** aids in the liver function as well as the detoxification.

**Hepatotoxic:** toxic to the liver.

**Hydrophilic:** easily mixes with or attracts water.

**Hydrophobic:** repels water.

**Hydrosol:** water byproduct of distillation; originally called hydrolat; historically known as flower waters.

**Hypertensive:** a substance that raises blood pressure.

**Hypnotic:** compels one to sleep.

**Hypoglycemic:** low blood sugar.

**Hypotensive:** a substance that reduces blood pressure.

**Immunity booster:** supports immune system function.

**Internal secretory structures:** cavities or ducts between cells within a plant that hold essential oils.

**Latin binomial:** Latin name identifying the genus and species of a plant.

**Lipophilic:** determines whether a substance is fat soluble.

**Lymphatic stimulant:** helps with cleaning the tissues in the lymphatic system.

**Maceration:** when flowers are soaked in hot oil to extract their essence.

**Mucolytic:** diminishes the thickness of mucus in the respiratory tract.

**Nervine:** strengthens the nervous system.

**Neurotonic:** tonic for the nervous system.

**Neurotoxic:** toxic to the nervous system.

**Oxidation:** alteration due to exposure to air; drying out.

**Photosensitization:** effect and damage that can occur on the skin after exposure to UV light.

**Photosynthesis:** process in which plants create food and oxygen.

**Phototoxicity:** a photosensitive substance applied to the skin and exposed to UV rays will result in skin damage and burning.

**Primary metabolites:** necessary components for plant growth and development such as amino acids and carbohydrates.

**Prophylactic:** prevents the spreading of disease.

**Rubefacient:** encourages blood circulation and causes redness in affected area.

**Secondary metabolites:** substances created for specific purposes, such as reproduction and protection. Essential oils are secondary metabolites.

**Secretory cells:** cells within a plant, such as ginger, that hold essential oils that must be broken to release the oil.

**Sedative:** produces a relaxing effect.

**Sensitization:** negative response the body has to a substance (rash, allergic reactions, etc.)

**Solvent extraction:** the use of solvents to remove certain plant tissue to gain access to essential oils.

**Stimulant:** a substance that increases the function of a system temporarily.

**Stomachic:** stimulates appetite and aids in digestion.

**Synergy:** a blend of two or more essential oils.

**Tonic:** supportive and restorative substance.

**Transpiration:** exchange of water vapor into the air and carbon dioxide into the plant.

**Uterine:** a tonic for the uterus.

**Volatile:** substance that moves from a liquid to a vapor.

**Vulnerary:** encourages the healing of damaged tissue.

## Professional Aromatherapy Associations

Alliance of International Aromatherapists
3000 South Jamaica Ct., Ste 145
Aurora, CO 80014
303-531-6377
www.alliance-aromatherapists.org

National Association for Holistic Aromatherapy
PO Box 27871
Raleigh, NC 27611-7871
919-894-0298
naha.org

International Federation of Professional
 Aromatherapists
82 Ashby Road
Hinckley, Leicestershire
LE10 1SN
United Kingdom
00 44 (0) 1455 637987
www.ifparoma.org

## Aromatherapy Education (in person and online)

American College of Healthcare Services
achs.edu

Aromahead Institute School of Essential Oil
 Studies
www.aromahead.com

Aromatic Wisdom Institute, School of Creative
 Aromatherapy
aromaticwisdominstitute.com

Ashi Therapy, School for Animal Aromatherapy and
 Botanical Studies
www.ashitherapy.com

Floracopeia
www.floracopeia.com

Institute of Holistic Phyto-Aromatherapy
authenticaromatherapyeducation.com

Institute of Integrative Aromatherapy
www.aroma-rn.com

*continued*

New York Institute of Aromatic Studies
nyioa.com

Stillpoint Studies
stillpointstudies.com

# References and Further Reading

AgriFarming. "Palmarosa Cultivation Information Guide." http://www.agrifarming.in/palmarosa-cultivation/. Accessed 2017.

Arctander, Steffen. *Perfume and Flavor Materials of Natural Origin*. Carol Stream, IL: Allured Publishing Corporation, 2008.

Arnica. "What Is Arnica Used For?" http://www.arnica.com/category/arnica-uses/. Accessed 2017.

AromaWeb. "Aromatherapy Bath Salts Recipe." https://www.aromaweb.com/recipes/bathsalts.asp. Accessed 2017.

———. "Essential Oil Shelf Life." http://www.aromaweb.com/articles/essentialoilshelflife.asp. Accessed 2017.

———. "Phototoxicity and Essential Oils." https://www.aromaweb.com/articles/phototoxicity-essential-oils.asp. Accessed 2017.

Axel, Richard, and Linda B. Buck. "Olfactory Receptor and Organization of Olfactory System." Nobel Peace Prize, 2004. http://www.nobelprize.org/nobel_prizes/medicine/laureates/2004/press.html.

Bakunas, C. D. "Distilling—How Old Is This Art?"

*Local Wines and Spirits*, February 8, 2011, WordPress. https://localwinecompany.wordpress.com/2011/02/08/distilling-how-old-is-this-art/. Accessed 2017.

Binns, Corey. "How We Smell." *Live Science*, May 22, 2006. http://www.livescience.com/10457-smell.html. Accessed 2017.

Bokelmann, Jean, MD. "What Is Endobiogeny?" Endobiogentic Integrative Medical Center. http://www.endobiogenic.com/Medical-Treatment-Definition-Pocatello-ID.html. Accessed 2017.

Browley, Cynthia, and Joy Musacchio. *Harvest and Distillation Experience*. Sedona, AZ: Stillpoint Studies, 2016.

Butje, Andrea. *The Heart of Aromatherapy: An Easy-to-Use Guide for Essential Oils*. Carlsbad, CA: Hay House, Inc., 2017.

Chard, Rose. *Carrier Oils and Their Role in Aromatherapy*. Raleigh, NC: National Association of Holistic Aromatherapy, 2016.

College of Pharmacy. "Show Globes." September 17, 2015, University of Arizona. http://www.pharmacy.arizona.edu/visitors/pharmacy-museum/show-globes. Accessed 2017.

Crow, David. *Sacred Smoke: The Magic and Medicine of Palo Santo*. Florecopeia Aromatic Treasures, 2012.

———. "Advanced Aromatherapy." Shift Network, Grass Valley, CA, 2016.

———. "HuaLu Aromatherapy." Florecopeia, Grass Valley, CA, 2016.

———. "Pharmacy of Flowers." Florecopeia, Grass Valley, CA, 2014.

Cupressaceae time line, Mezoanic era. https://www.britannica.com/plant/gymnosperm.

Davis, Patricia. *Aromatherapy: An A–Z.* New York: Barnes & Noble, 1988.

Delevorya, T. "Gymnosperm." *Encyclopaedia Britannica.* https://www.britannica.com/plant/gymnosperm. Accessed 2017.

Denker, Joel. "'Moon of the Faith': A History of the Apricot and Its Many Pleasures." *The Salt,* NPR. June 14, 2016. http://www.npr.org/sections/thesalt/2016/06/14/481932829/moon-of-the-faith-a-history-of-the-apricot-and-its-many-pleasures. Accessed 2017.

Edens Garden. "This or That: All About Frankincense Carterii, Frereana, and Serrata." April 22, 2016. https://www.edensgarden.com/blogs/news/115923396-this-or-that-all-about-frankincense-carterii-frereana-and-serrata. Accessed 2017.

Ehrlich, Steven D., NMD. "Peppermint." University of Maryland Medical Center, July 6, 2014. http://www.umm.edu/health/medical/altmed/herb/peppermint. Accessed 2017.

*Encyclopaedia Britannica.* "Geranium." https://www.britannica.com/plant/geranium-plant-genus-Geranium. Accessed 2017.

Encyclopedia of Life. "*Prunus amygdalus*/Sweet Almond." http://eol.org/pages/231567/overview. Accessed 2017.

———. "*Vitis vinifera*/European Grape." http://eol.org/pages/582304/overview. Accessed 2017.

Essential Oil University. "Essential Oil Myths." https://essentialoils.org/news/eo_myths. Accessed 2017.

Foster, Jane. "Gut Feelings: Bacteria and the Brain." *Cerebrum,* July 1, 2013. https://www.ncbi.nlm.nih.gov/pmc/articles/PMC3788166/. Accessed 2017.

Franzen, Harald. "Plants Attract Enemy's Enemies to Survive." *Scientific American,* March 16, 2001. https://www.scientificamerican.com/article/plants-attract-enemys-ene/. Accessed 2017.

Frolova, Victoria. "Speaking Perfume: A–Z of Common Fragrance Descriptions." Bois de Jasmin, February 3, 2012. http://boisdejasmin.com/2012/02/speaking-perfume-a-z-of-common-fragrance-descriptions.html. Accessed 2017.

Fulcher, Liz. "AWP 024: Safe Aromatherapy for Children." Aromatic Wisdom Institute, July 21, 2016 (podcast). http://aromaticwisdominstitute.com/024/.

Gardener, Z., and M. McGuffin, eds. *American Herbal Products Association's Botanical Safety Handbook,* 2nd ed. Boca Raton, FL: CRC Press, 2013.

Gattefossé, René-Maurice. *Gattefossé's Aromatherapy.* Edited by Robert Tisserand. Essex, UK: C. W. Daniel Company, 1993 (Originally published Paris: Giradeau & Cie, 1937).

Goldbaum, Kate. "What Is the Oldest Tree in the World?" *Live Science,* August 23, 2016. http://

www.livescience.com/29152-oldest-tree-in
-world.html. Accessed 2017.

Grieve, M. "Chamomiles." Botanical. http://www
.botanical.com/botanical/mgmh/c/chammo49
.html. Accessed 2017.

Gumbel, D. *Principles of Holistic Therapy with Herbal
Essences.* Brussels: Haug International, 1993, 204.

Hardin, Jesse Wolf. "Plant Totems: Identifying Our
Most Personal Herbal Ally." The Medicine
Woman's Roots. http://bearmedicineherbals
.com/plant-totems-identifying-our-most
-personal-herbal-ally-by-jesse-wolf-hardin.html.
Accessed 2017.

Isaac, Michael. *A Historical Atlas of Oman.* New
York: Rosen Publishing Group, 2004, 14.

Keville, K., and M. Green. *Aromatherapy: A
Complete Guide to the Healing Art.* Berkeley,
CA: Crossing Press, 2009.

Kinsey, T. Beth. "Cestrum nocturnum—Night-
blooming Jasmine." Wild Life of Hawaii. http://
wildlifeof
hawaii.com/flowers/967/cestrum-nocturnum
-night-blooming-jasmine/. Accessed 2017.

Largest Fastest Smartest. "Animals with the Best
Sense of Smell in the World." January 18, 2008.
http://largestfastestsmartest.co.uk/animals
-with-the-best-sense-of-smell-in-the-world/.
Accessed 2017.

Lawless, Julia. *Aromatherapy and the Mind.* London:
Thorsons, 1994.

———. *The Illustrated Encyclopedia of Essential
Oils: The Complete Guide to the Use of Oils
in Aromatherapy and Herbalism.* Bath, UK:
Mustard, 1995.

Li, Q., M. Kobayashi, Y. Wakayama, H. Inagaki, M.
Katsumata, Y. Hirata, K. Hirata, T. Shimizu, T.
Kawada, B. J. Park, T. Ohira, T. Kagawa, and Y.
Miyazaki. "Effect of Phytoncide from Trees on
Human Natural Killer Cell Function." PubMed,
October 2009. https://www.ncbi.nlm.nih.gov/
pubmed/20074458. Accessed 2017.

Long, Jim. "Down to Earth: The Real Curry Plant."
*Mother Earth Living*, June/July 2003. http://
www.motherearthliving.com/gardening/the
-real-curry-plant?pageid=2#PageContent2.
Accessed 2017.

Matthews, Susan E. "5 Animals with an
Extraordinary Sense of Smell." *Popular Science*,
May 9, 2013. http://www.popsci.com/science/
article/2013-05/five-feats-smell#page-4.
Accessed 2017.

McDermott, Annette. "Doctrine of Signatures."
Love to Know. http://herbs.lovetoknow.com/
doctrine-signatures. Accessed 2017.

McMahon, Christopher. "Neroli." White Lotus
Aromatics. http://www.whitelotusaromatics.
com/newsletters/neroli. Accessed 2017.

Mojay, Gabriel. *Aromatherapy for Healing the Spirit:
A Guide to Restoring Emotional and Mental
Balance through Essential Oils.* London: Gaia,
2005.

Moldenauer, Leslie. "Move over 1,8 Cineole . . . a

review of essential oils that provide respiratory support for kids," October 26, 2017. https://www.lifeholistically.com. Accessed 2017.

Nesmith, Retha. "Can Essential Oils Be Ingested?" *Plant Therapy*, January 14, 2015. https://www.planttherapy.com/blog/2014/01/14/can-essential-oils-be-ingested/. Accessed 2017.

Orloff, Judith. "The Health Benefits of Tears." *Psychology Today*, July 27, 2010, Sussex Publishers, LLC. https://www.psychologytoday.com/blog/emotional-freedom/201007/the-health-benefits-tears. Accessed 2017.

Osborn, David K. "The Four Humors." Greek Medicine. http://www.greekmedicine.net/b_p/Four_Humors.html. Accessed 2017.

Park, B. J., Y. Tsunetsugu, T. Kasetani, T. Kagawa, and Y. Miyazaki. "The Physiological Effects of Shinrin-yoku (Taking in the Forest Atmosphere or Forest Bathing): Evidence from Field Experiments in 24 Forests Across Japan." PubMed, January 2010. https://www.ncbi.nlm.nih.gov/pubmed/19568835. Accessed 2017.

Parker, Susan M. *Power of the Seed: Your Guide to Oils for Health & Beauty*. Los Angeles: Process, 2015.

Parks, Christine. "Camellia Sinensis—Backyard Tea." American Camellias Society. https://www.americancamellias.com/care-culture-resources/the-camellia-family/camellia-sinensis-backyard-tea. Accessed 2017.

Plant & Soil Sciences Library. "Transpiration: Water Movement Through Plants." *Plant &* http://passel.unl.edu/pages/informationmodule.php?idinformationmodule=1092853841&topicorder=6. Accessed 2017.

Plant Science 4 U. "Primary and Secondary Metabolites." http://www.plantscience4u.com/2013/02/primary-and-secondary-metabolites.html#.WOkUodLyuM8. Accessed 2017.

Power, Joie, PhD. "Lavender Essential Oil." The Aromatherapy School. http://www.aromatherapy-school.com/aromatherapy-schools/aromatherapy-articles/essential-oil-monograph-lavender.html. Accessed 2017.

Prance, Ghillean, and Mark Nesbitt, eds. *The Cultural History of Plants*. New York: Routledge, 2005.

Pressimone, Jennifer. *JennScents Holistic Aromatherapy Comprehensive Guide*. Clearmont, FL: JennScents, Inc., 2015.

Price, Shirley. *Practical Aromatherapy: How to Use Essential Oils to Restore Vitality*. London: Thorsons, 1983.

PubChem. "Sclareol." June 24, 2005, National Center for Biotechnology Information. https://pubchem.ncbi.nlm.nih.gov/compound/Sclareol. Accessed 2017.

Reza, Shamim. "Plant Allelopathy." Permaculture, January 21, 2016. https://permaculturenews.org/2016/01/21/plant-allelopathy/. Accessed 2017.

Rhind, J. P. *Essential Oils: A Handbook for*

*Aromatherapy Practice*. London: Singing Dragon, 2012.

Richardson, Jill. "A Plant Enemy's Enemy." *Science News for Students*, April 3, 2013. https://www.sciencenewsforstudents.org/article/plant-enemy%E2%80%99s-enemy. Accessed 2017.

Roberts, Nancy. "Avoid Scents That Attract Bees." *Courier-Post*, May 4, 2015, http://www.courierpostonline.com/story/life/home-garden/2015/05/04/avoid-scents-attract-bees/26877045/. Accessed 2017.

Rose, Jeanne. *The Aromatherapy Book: Applications & Inhalations*. San Francisco, CA: North Atlantic Books, 1992.

Schnaubelt, Kurt, PhD. *The Healing Intelligence of Essential Oils: The Science of Advanced Aromatherapy*. Rochester, VT: Healing Arts Press, 2011.

Science Museum's History of Medicine. "Doctrine of Signatures." http://www.sciencemuseum.org.uk/broughttolife/techniques/doctrine. Accessed 2017.

Seed Guides. "Grapeseed Oil Benefits, Uses, Side Effects, Facts and Information." http://www.seedguides.info/grapeseed-oil/. Accessed 2017.

Shutes, Jade. *Aromatic Scholars*. Chapel Hill, NC: The New York Institute of Aromatic Studies, 2017.

———. *Foundations of Aromatherapy*. Chapel Hill, NC: The New York Institute of Aromatic Studies, 2016.

———. *How to Pronounce Latin Names of Aromatic Plants* (video). Chapel Hill, NC: The New York Institute of Aromatic Studies, 2017. https://vimeo.com/169378598.

Shutes, Jade, and Cathy Skipper. *French Aromatherapy*. Chapel Hill, NC: The New York Institute of Aromatic Studies, 2016.

Stansbury, Jillian. "Plant Intelligence: A Philosophical Discourse on Cognitive Awareness in Plants." Battle Ground Healing Arts. http://battlegroundhealingarts.com/articles/plant-intelligence-a-philosophical-discourse-on-cognitive-awareness-in-plants/. Accessed 2017.

———. *Jill Stansbury*. Homestead, 2016. http://www.jillstansbury.net/. Accessed 2017.

Super Herbs. "Lemongrass." http://www.superbherbs.net/lemongrass.htm. Accessed 2017.

Tea Forté. "The Secret History of Jasmine Tea." https://www.teaforte.com/tealiving/the-secret-history-of-jasmine-tea/. Accessed 2017.

Tisserand, Robert. "Frankincense Essential Oil and Cancer." http://roberttisserand.com/2015/03/frankincense-essential-oil-and-cancer/. Accessed 2017. Tisserand, April 22, 2011. http://roberttisserand.com/2011/04/gattefosses-burn/. Accessed 2017.

———. "Is Clary Sage Oil Estrogenic." http://roberttisserand.com/2010/04/is-clary-sage-oil-estrogenic/. April 2010. Accessed 2017.

———. "Learn More/Drop Size." Tisserand Institute.

http://tisserandinstitute.org/learn-more/drop
-size. Accessed 2017.

———. "Learn More/Topical Safety Guidelines."
http://tisserandinstitute.org/learn-more/
topical-safety-guidelines/. Accessed 2017.

Tisserand, Robert B. *The Art of Aromatherapy*, rev.
ed. Rochester, VT, Healing Arts Press 1990.

Tisserand, Robert, and Rodney Young. *Essential Oil
Safety: A Guide for Health Care Professionals*,
2nd ed. Edinburgh: Elsevier, 2014.

TopTropicals. "The Bearer of an Ideal Fragrance."
https://toptropicals.com/html/toptropicals/
articles/trees/cananga.htm. Accessed 2017.

Waksmundzka-Hajnos, Monika, and Joseph Sherma,
eds. *High Performance Liquid Chromatography
in Phytochemical Analysis*. Boca Raton, FL: CRC
Press, 2010, 103.

War, A. R., M. G. Paulraj, T. Ahmad, A. A. Buhroo, B.
Hussain, S. Ignacimuthu, et al. "Mechanisms
of Plant Defense Against Insect Herbivores."
*Plant Signaling and Behavior* 7, no. 10 (2012):
1306–20. doi: 10.4161/psb.21663. https://www.
ncbi.nlm.nih.gov/pmc/articles/PMC3493419/.

Web MD. "Marjoram." http://www.webmd.com/
vitamins-supplements/ingredientmono-563

-marjoram.aspx?activeingredientid=563.
Accessed 2017.

Webb, Mark. "CO2 Extracts." Brisbane, Queensland,
Australia, 2017.

———. "Bush Sense: The Therapeutic, Spiritual, and
Shamanic Uses of Australian Essential Oils and
Aromatic Compounds." NAHA Conference,
Salt Lake City, UT, 2016.

Welch, Craig. "Provence's Legendary Lavender and
Olives Threatened by a Changing Climate."
*National Geographic*, December 11, 2015.
http://news.nationalgeographic
.com/2015/12/151211-paris-climate-lavender
-wine-olives-truffles-provence/. Accessed 2017.

Williams, Amanda. "Why Do Bees Need Nectar and
Pollen?" Buzz About Bees. http://www.buzz
aboutbees.net/why- do- bees- need- nectar- and-
pollen.html. Accessed 2017.

Wood, Matthew. "The Doctrine of Signatures."
NaturaSophia, March 27, 2011. http://www
.naturasophia.com/Signatures.html. Accessed
2017.

Worwood, Valerie Ann. *The Complete Book of
Essential Oils and Aromatherapy*. San Rafael,
CA: New World Library, 1991.

# ACKNOWLEDGMENTS

To all those who have shown me the stepping stones of essential oils, plant wisdom, and the overlapping wisdom between the world seen and unseen; pioneers, guides, and teachers such as David Crow, Jade Shutes, Madeleine Kerkhof-Knapp Hayes, Joy Musacchio, Cynthia Brownley, Gabriel Mojay, Robert Tisserand, Mark Webb, Jeanne Rose, Jane Buckle, Kurt Schnaubelt, Valerie Ann Wormwood, Liz Fulcher, Andrea Butje, Mindy Green, Rose Chard, Ann Harmon, Marge Clark, John Black, Cathy Skipper, Kelly Holland Azzaro, Roxana Villa, Amy Emnet, Robert Pappas, Jean Bokelmann, Chris Burder, Nancy Cyr, Ester Ng, and many others. To Theresa Cangialosi, Michelle Cohen, and Donna Audia.

To every educator in aromatherapy who does due diligence in keeping in view the respect of plant knowledge and powerful medicine. To the "grandfathers" and "grandmothers" in the plant education world: Your deep wisdom far exceeds the fast-paced Internet nibbles people eat up. Thank you Ann Treistman, Aurora Bell, and Tracy Vega. To Mark and Lance, and especially to Sedona, your help was invaluable. To Sally and Lee. And last, to all those who are new to aromatherapy and essential oils. May you find your introduction to the grand wisdom and power of essential oils to be fulfilling, deeply self-empowering, and awakening. May you find more of yourself in this aromatic journey.

Page 226: Chart modified from *Essential Oil Safety*, Second Edition, Tisserand, R. and Young, R., Table 4.6/Chapter 4, page 48, Copyright 2014, reprinted with permission from Elsevier.

Page 228: Chart compiled in collaboration with Robert Tisserand (Tisserand Institute) and Jade Shutes (New York Institutes of Aromatic Studies), used by permission.

Pages 229–31: Charts reproduced with modifications from Jade Shutes (New York Institutes of Aromatic Studies), by permission.

**All photographs by Cher Kaufmann, unless otherwise indicated.**

Page 20: © Grisha Bruev / shutterstock.com; page 22: © photogal / shuttersock.com; page 34: Esther Ng; page 38: © Alin Brotea / shutterstock.com; pages 39, 40, 41 right, 42, 74, 77: Robert Baker; page 41 Ieft: © rukxstockphoto / shutterstock.com; page 47: © Lorenzo Sala / shutterstock.com; page 57 top: © Polina Shestakova / shutterstock.com; page 57 bottom: © Yomka / shutterstock.com; pages 60, 160: © joloei / shutterstock.com; page 64: © Irina Bg / shutterstock.com; page 73: © Irma eyewink / shutterstock.com; page 76: © Joop Snijder Photography / shutterstock.com; page 82: © KosmosIII / shutterstock.com; page 95: © knape / iStockPhoto.com; page 98: Bria Cleaver; page 120 top: © Viktory Panchenko / shutterstock.com; pages 123, 207: © grafvision / shutterstock.com; pages 126 right, 162 center: © Correcaminos112 / shutterstock.com; page 128: © CHANSIP SILARAT / shutterstock.com; page 129: © Juan Aunion / shutterstock.com; pages 130, 157, 257: © Ivana Vrnoga / shutterstock.com; page 132: © janaph / shutterstock.com; pages 133, 156: © JSOBHATIS16899 / shutterstock.com; pages 137, 162 right: © Stephen Orsillo / shutterstock.com; pages 138 top, 168: © Iness_la_luz / shutterstock.com; pages 138 bottom, 169: © Alaa AbuMadi / shutterstock.com; page 139: © Zurainy Zain / shutterstock.com; page 142: © John A. Cameron / shutterstock.com; page 144: © Maros Markovic / shutterstock.com; page 145: © Sinisa Glisic / shutterstock.com; page 154: © iomis / shutterstock.com; page 159: © phetsamay philavanh / shutterstock.com; page 161: © ntdanai / shutterstock.com; page 162 left: © alessandro0770 / iStockPhoto.com; page 164: © jakubtravelphoto / shutterstock.com; page 170: © RukiMedia / shutterstock.com; page 173: © Passakorn Umpommaha / shutterstock.com; page 179: © Sakda tiew / shutterstock.com; page 180: © anat chant / shutterstock.com; page 192: © Cenz07 / shutterstock.com; pages 196, 274: © Peter Turner Photography / shutterstock.com; page 197: © Anna Ok / shutterstock.com; page 203: © DSLucas / shutterstock.com; page 206: © ZigZag Mountain Art / shutterstock.com; page

# INDEX

Frustration Soother (recipe), 263
Fulcher, Liz, 56, 105
fungicide, 135
fungus, 99, 105, 135, 196, 243, 258
furanocoumarins, 62

**G**

Galen, 135
Galland, Antoine, 250
gamma linoleic acid, 240
gas, 84; and chamomile, 155; and children, 230; and ginger, 208; and patchouli, 138; and peppermint, 140; and rosemary, 148; and sweet fennel, 124, 230; and sweet marjoram, 167
gas chromatography (GC), 32, 62, 63
gastrointestinal tract (GI), 83
Gattefossé, René-Maurice, 27, 28
GC. *See* gas chromatography
gels, 243–44
Geraniacaea, 159
geranial, as aldehyde, 60
geranium. *See* rose geranium
ginger, 48, 207–10; and Muscle Relief Blend (recipe), 167; and After Shower/After Workout (recipe), 182; and alertness, 123; and bloating, 84; and calm, 85; and cancer, 200; and children, 231; and Cough Soother Room Diffuser (recipe), 264; and depression, 87; and Desert Sunset (recipe), 272; and digestion, 121, 179; and Earth and Sky (recipe), 274; and End-of-Day Relaxing Blend (recipe), 267; and grounding, 87; and massage, 122, 124; and Meditation Blend (recipe), 202; and Memory and Study (recipe), 262; and nausea, 200,

230; as sesquiterpenes, 59; and Spicy Citrus Feel-Good Personal Inhaler (recipe), 187; and spirituality, 123; and Spot Treatment Sore Muscle/Joint Rub (recipe), 191; and sprain care salve (recipe), 269; and Sunshine Zest (recipe), 236; and Warm My Toes (recipe), 123; and Warming Bath (recipe), 270; and warmth, 81, 270
glandular trichomes, 47
Goethe, Johann von, 45
Goldbaum, Kate, 33
Good Morning Wake-Up (recipe), 141
Good Night Open Heart Emotion Soother (recipe), 160
Graminaea, 210, 213, 215
grapefruit, 181–83; and Air Freshener (recipe), 136; and Citrus Rosemary Air Purifier (recipe), 185; and clear head, 85; and depression, 87; and Good Morning Wake-up (recipe), 141; and harmony, 123; and nootkatone, 60; and phototoxicity, 178; and Spicy Citrus Feel-Good Personal Inhaler (recipe), 187; and Sunshine Zest (recipe), 236
grapeseed oil, 246, 253–54
Greeks: and "Doctrine of Signatures," 45; and aromatic plants, 25, 26; and chamomile, 154; and ginger, 208; and laurel, 135; and lemon, 184; and patchouli, 137; and peppermint, 140; and pine, 142; and rosemary, 147; and sesame, 250; and sweet marjoram, 166; and the four humors, 65
Green, Mindy, 70
Grieves, 154
grounding: and base notes, 232; and

frankincense, 198; and Frustration Soother (recipe), 263; and ginger, 87, 208, 209; and Grounding and Calming Blend (recipe), 211; and patchouli, 139, 236; and vetiver, 87, 209, 210
Grounding and Calming Blend (recipe), 211
Gumbel, D., on lemongrass, 215

**H**

hair follicle, 80
hair: and carrier oils, 105; and cedarwood, 197; and cistus, 131; and coconut oil, 249; and dermis layer, 80; and Hair Tonic (recipe), 266; and hair-nutritive carriers, 247; and jojoba, 249, 250; and mandarin, 186; and rose geranium, 160; and rose, 171; and rosemary, 148; and Scalp Tonic (recipe), 148; and sweet almond oil, 252; and sweet orange, 189; and ylang-ylang, 173
Hair Tonic (recipe), 266
Harmon, Ann, 52
Haskell, David George, 33
Hayes, Madeleine Kerkhof-Knapp, 31, 244
healing, wounds: and bergamot, 179; and calendula herbal oil, 258; and chamomile, 155; and cistus, 131; and eucalyptus, 132; and foraha oil, 255; and frankincense, 199; and gamma linoleic acid, 241; and grapeseed oil, 254; and Jean Valnet, 28; and ketones, 60; and lavender, 99, 164; and palmarosa, 216; and rosemary, 147; and vetiver, 210; and water-based remedies, 244; and Wound-Healing First-Aid Gel Spray (recipe), 130